PSYCHIATRY MADE RIDICULOUSLY SIMPLE

by

William V. Good, M.D.

Professor and Chairman, Department of Ophthalmology
University of Cincinnati College of Medicine
Director, Abrahamson Pediatric Eye Institute
Cincinnati Children's Hospital

and

Jefferson E. Nelson, M.D.

Private Practice
Fellow, American Psychiatric Association
Austin, Texas

Art by Don P. Bridge, D.D.S.

MedMaster, Inc., Miami

ISBN # 0-940780-22-4

Made in the United States of America

Published by
MedMaster, Inc.
P.O. Box 640028
Miami, FL 33164

Third Printing, 1987; *Fourth Printing,* 1987; *Fifth Printing,* 1990; *Sixth Print-
ing,* 1991; *Seventh Printing,* 1992; *Eighth Printing,* 1993; *Ninth Printing,* 1995;
Tenth Printing, 1997; *Eleventh Printing,* 1999.

DEDICATION

TO LAURIE, BENJAMIN, SAMUEL, PHYLLIS, ALEX, AND JACK.

TABLE OF CONTENTS

PREFACE

Although humor is used in this book to highlight diagnostic findings, it is not our intent to laugh at people with psychiatric problems. On the contrary, we hope that reading this book will enable you to help and understand patients better.

Where appropriate, we have integrated the DSM III (Diagnostic and Statistical Manual of Mental Disorders, Third Edition, American Psychiatric Association) into the text. For lists of diagnostic criteria and a complete review of the psychiatric nomenclature, the reader is referred to this reference manual.

We are indebted to Susan Domaschk for her help in preparing this book.

PREFACE TO THE SECOND EDITION

In the four years since this book was last revised a number of important events have occurred in psychiatry. Some of these include: the introduction of the DSM—III—R (Diagnostic and Statistical Manual of Mental Disorders, Third Edition, Revised, American Psychiatric Association, 1987); the release of several new psychotropic medications such as fluoxetine, clomipramine, and clozapine; research findings on the efficacy of certain types of psychotherapy; and a heightened focus on the psychological trauma and disability resulting from abuse, particularly sexual abuse.

We have attempted to engage the reader in a 'conversation' throughout this book. The 'psychiatrist' we address may be a medical student, psychiatric resident, or graduate student in psychology, social work or other field. The context we imply is usually a medical one but we believe the information contained here is applicable and pertinent in a wide range of mental health settings.

PREFACE TO THE THIRD EDITION

The DSM is now in its fourth edition (Diagnostic and Statistical Manual of Mental Disorders, Fourth Edition, American Psychiatric Association, 1994, DSM IV). Fluoxetine has been followed by three related medications, fluvoxamine, sertraline and paroxetine, creating a new class of antidepressants, the SSRI's (selective serotonin reuptake inhibitors). The terms organic mental syndrome and organic brain syndrome have been deleted from the DSM IV to underscore the idea that all psychiatric disorders have physiological components. We hope this book will continue to provide a concise and practical guide to our field.

CHAPTER 1. INTRODUCTION

Contrary to popular opinion, psychiatrists deal with topics other than sex. What could be more important than sex? The psychiatrist deals with many varieties of mental dysfunction. One can appreciate this simply by reviewing some of the common terms in psychiatry:

Affect: Psychiatrists are always interested in how a patient feels at a particular time. Sadness, anger, happiness, and irritation are all examples of affects. The type of affect, its appropriateness to the situation, its stability, and its intensity are important diagnostically (see Mood).

Akathisia: A state of motor restlessness, commonly seen as a side effect of anti-psychotic drugs. The patient seems unable to sit still and usually is very troubled by this symptom.

Attention: The ability to concentrate on a task.

Autistic: This term refers to modes of behavior in which the patient disregards his environment in a pervasive way appearing to respond to internal stimuli only.

Blocking: Thought processes stop for emotional reasons. This commonly occurs in grand rounds presentations.

Capitation: Placing a monetary value for purposes of insurance reimbursement on a disease, usually expressed as a fraction. Numerator = value of disease (usually expressed in cents); denominator = piece of body under consideration (e.g. limbic system); subdenominator = time period of insurance (usually expressed in decades or centuries).

Carve Out: An end run around capitation.

Catatonia: This is a state of stupor with alteration in motor functioning. It may occur in psychosis and mood disorders but is also seen in certain neurological conditions. House staff may become catatonic after being on call for 48 hours straight.

Circumstantiality: Too much digression precedes communication of central idea.

Clanging: Thoughts occur in sequence because of the way words sound, not because of content.

Compulsion: This is the need to perform an act repetitively. People with obsessions and compulsions usually understand that the behavior is abnormal, are distressed by the behavior, but feel unable to do anything to change it.

Confabulation: Spontaneously making up facts that can't be remembered. Commonly a sign of alcohol-induced dementia or similar disorder.

Conversion: This refers to a loss of neurologic functioning in the absence of a documented central nervous system lesion(s).

Countertransference: Inappropriate feelings that doctors have for their patients. By this we mean feelings that get in the way of proper patient care.

Cyclothymia: This term refers to alternating periods of elation and depression which characterize a specific mood disorder.

Defense Mechanisms: These are aspects of one's personality (specifically of the ego) that help combat specific uncomfortable or unwanted feelings or thoughts.

Defense mechanisms include reaction formation, denial, repression, identification and others. These are explained later in a clinical example.

Delirium: This is often a reversible, acute alteration in brain function with disturbance of consciousness and thinking. See Chapter 2 for more details.

Delusion: This is a false belief neither based on reality, nor culturally derived, and not altered by reasonable evidence to the contrary. For example, a patient tells you that the IRS is out to get him because he hasn't paid his income tax. If he doesn't have a job or income, he has a delusion!

Dementia: This is (usually) irreversible loss of memory and cognitive functioning. More on this can be found in Chapter 2.

Depression: A mental state of sadness, usually accompanied by low self-esteem, self-reproach and other signs and symptoms.

Dystonic Reaction: As a side effect of phenothiazines and other antipsychotics, and a neurologic condition, dystonia refers to spasmodic muscular contractions, especially of the neck, face, and back.

DSM IV: Diagnostic and Statistical Manual of Mental Disorders, Fourth Edition, published by the American Psychiatric Association, 1994.

Ego: This is a metaphorical concept used by Freud to describe those parts of the human psyche that deal with reality (e.g., intellect, perception, memory, defense mechanisms). The term is used inaccurately in common parlance to mean an inflated sense of self-worth.

Flight of Ideas: Thoughts occur in rapid succession and may be incoherent. This is seen most commonly in the manic phase of bipolar disorder.

Formication: This is the feeling that insects are crawling on your skin. It is a type of hallucination caused by cocaine and delirium tremens.

Hallucination: This is the perception of a sensory stimulus in the absence of any sensory stimulus. Hallucinations come in all sensory varieties.

Id: This term refers to the part of the mind hypothesized by Freud to contain inherent aggressive and sexual drives.

Ideas of Reference: This is when the patient feels that specific events (like television shows or the actions of other people) refer directly to the patient. They are focal delusions.

Illusion: This is the misperception of a sensory stimulus.

Loose Associations: Loose associations are not organizations like the AMA or the Elk's Club. The term actually refers to a process of thinking in which ideas in the stream of thought have no relation to each other. "Star Trek is my favorite TV program, I like Spock the best, the traffic lights are red and green and amber is in the middle and Pegasus was a flying horse" is an example of loose associations from a young schizophrenic patient. If it makes sense to you, you must have been on call last night.

Managed Care: Managed lack of care.

Mania: A mood characterized by elation and increased activity (see Chapter 2).

Mood: Pervasive feelings that are experienced internally. The external expression of the feeling is termed *affect.*

Neurosis: In psychiatry, this is a term afforded patients in relatively good psychological health. In other medical fields, the term is pejorative. Theoretically, the term refers to problems such as depression, anxiety, and conversion reactions which are the result of intrapsychic conflict. We can't define the term further, because we would have to bring up the topic of sex again.

Obsession: This is an idea or thought that constantly intrudes into consciousness.

Orientation: Understanding one's environment, in terms of time, place, and person.

Paranoia: This is the delusional feeling that people are out to get you.

Personality Disorder: Characteristic, stable and maladaptive ways of behaving. See Chapter 12 for discussion of types of personality disorders.

Psychobabble: Psychiatric jargon.

Psychosis: This term usually refers to a problem in which the patient has lost touch with reality. Clinically speaking, it refers to patients suffering from delusions, hallucinations, and significantly disordered thought processes.

Reality Testing: The ability to appreciate what one's environment is really like.

Schizophrenia: A mental illness causing hallucinations, delusions, and loose associations (see Chapter 2).

Superego: Conscience. Freud coined this term.

Transference: This is the misperceiving of a person in the present as having the qualities of someone from the patient's past life. This distortion may be gross and almost transparent, as in figure 1, or it may be very subtle. It would be worse pathology to think the two people are the same. In this case, the transference is psychotic or delusional.

A long time ago, a neurologist by the name of Sigmund Freud became interested in neurological conditions for which there seemed to be no sound neurologic or neuropathologic findings. His curiosity about these patients with hysterical conversion symptoms led him to attempt hypnosis on them. He discovered that such patients frequently repressed (forgot) traumatic childhood events or memories. As adults, they re-enacted these repressed memories in conflict-symptom constellations; that is, lived out and repeated these memories in maladaptive ways in an effort to master the childhood experience.

The word *conflict,* is one that psychiatrists kick around a lot. It's not a conflict of the Arab-Israeli variety, but rather one that occurs in an individual's mind. When a repressed wish meets with a prohibition against the wish (and these prohibitions are intra-psychic), then a conflict develops. A third-year medical student, anxious to kick up his heels on Friday evening, usually shakes hands with conflict when his intern or resident suggests that they go see an interesting patient. (Fig. 2).

The conflict is that the medical student would like to slug the resident but is obliged to hold back. To strike the resident would be relatively uncivilized and contrary to what the average student has learned about dealing with other human beings. How does the psyche deal with the wish and the prohibition against the wish, both which are in "conflict" with each other? This is where defense mechanisms often come into play. The student may say, "Fantastic, I love seeing inter-

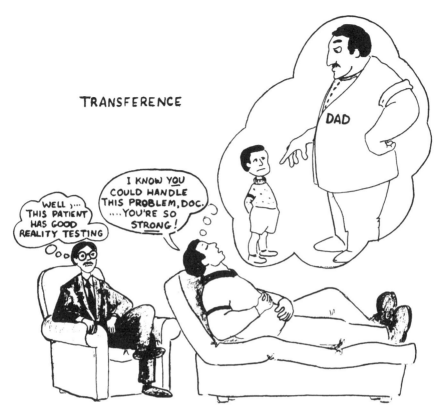

Fig 1. Patient having transference; doctor having delusion.

esting patients." This reversal of anger is termed *reaction formation*. On the other hand, he may glumly accompany the resident, and a few years later pull the same stunt on his medical student. This would be termed *identification with the aggressor!* If the medical student wants to slug the resident, raises his arm and fist, and then develops a paralysis of the arm, this is a *conversion* symptom. A somatic symptom is now being used to defend against the wish to slug a superior. If the medical student were hypnotized, this buried aggressive wish would most likely be brought to the surface.

You must be wondering why hypnosis isn't the treatment of choice, then, for all of these intrapsychic disorders. Although Freud found that hypnosis could frequently uncover the buried conflict and memory, he found that psychoanalysis, a technique that involves a detailed interaction between patient and physician, was more effective in treating emotional diseases. He discovered that the best way to cure conversion or hysterical symptoms was to unravel, decode, and understand the myriad of defense mechanisms and resistances in his patients. These resistances, defense mechanisms, and transferences are typically more complex than our scheme above. By the way, couches for patients came into

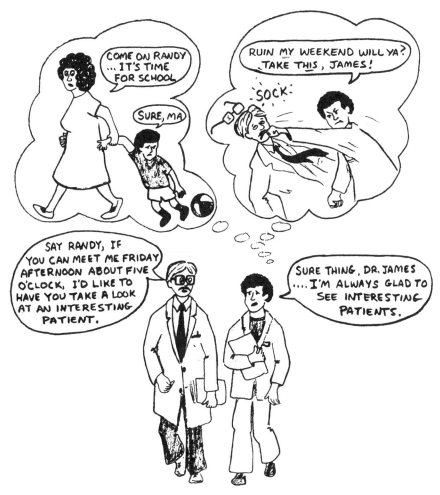

Fig. 2. Conflict between wanting to slug the resident and holding back; transference of mother-child and resident-student roles.

vogue to facilitate transference, and the psychoanalyst moved behind the pa tient's head for the same reason. He also could yawn, stretch, or fall asleep, without the patient's knowing! Modern transformations of Freud's psychoanalytic technique and theory include psychoanalysis, couch and all, and psychotherapy, which involves a face to face encounter of patient with therapist. Today, psychotherapies may be broadly categorized as dynamic (focused on resolution of intrapsychic conflict) or cognitive-behavioral (focused on changing distorted and maladaptive thoughts, feelings and behaviors).

Here we have perhaps the most important distinction between psychiatry and other medical subspecialities. In other fields, diseases are considered as static entities. The patient "*has* a case of pneumonia" for which he will be treated with a specific and quantifiable dose of penicillin. Or, the patient *had* an M.I. at 10:20 AM at the age of 46. This static model of disease usually serves medicine very well, but not psychiatry. Psychopathology in psychiatry is viewed as illness that develops gradually over a period of time. A bio-psychosocial model is used to account for the development of psychiatric illnesses. This theory takes into consideration the individual's physical endowment, his psychological endowment, and cultural and/or social factors in the development of his illness. The interplay of all three over time accounts for the development of psychiatric (and even medical) illness.

During the initial evaluation of the patient the psychiatrist takes the history and performs a mental status examination (see Chapter 2). The psychiatrist must evaluate the patient's symptoms and signs and get historical information from the biopsychosocial perspective to adequately evaluate the patient. The patient's personal and family history of illnesses as well as life traumas are particularly relevant. The initial diagnostic impression will lead to a treatment plan addressing the need for psychotropic medication (bio), psychotherapy (psycho), and social interventions (social).

When a patient comes to see a psychiatrist for intra-psychic or inter-personal problems and is not suffering from one of the major psychoses or mood disorders that will be discussed later, he is usually invited to participate in a psychotherapy *process*. This is literally the development of wide ranging interactions between the patient and his psychiatrist over a period of time. During these interactions, defense mechanisms, transference phenomena, and resistances to exploring difficult subjects for the patient may arise. These are interpreted by the psychiatrist to the patient to help the patient unravel the mysteries of his own life. The principles are sound and sensible. Patience is the order of the day. A busy neurologist working in the emergency room whose patient presents with a neurotic conversion disorder may not understand this. All he wants is a cure in the next 24 hours! Any self respecting psychiatrist will say that he and his patient need time. Newer therapies are often limited to 8-12 visits, however!

This brings up another aspect of the role of psychiatry in the practice of medicine. Although psychiatrists are geared to manage mental illness, they are also called upon to help negotiate other difficult situations that may arise in busy medical or hospital practices. Difficulties between nursing staff, physicians, or administrative personnel can be a part of the psychiatrist's domain. Most psychiatrists have special training in management of interpersonal conflict and group dynamics even when psychopathology is not of primary importance. Unfortunately, sometimes psychiatrists are asked to function as sanitation engineers in the hospital. "Get this patient off my back" is an occasional request made by referring physician to a psychiatrist. "This patient wants to sue me, make him stop feeling that way" is a psychiatrist-as-brainwasher view of the specialty.

As a rule of thumb, a psychiatrist should become involved in a psychologically difficult or psychologically related case early in the management of the case. In the work-up of conversion disorders, the psychiatric diagnosis should not be a diagnosis of exclusion. Early psychiatric intervention helps prevent the patient from feeling that he has been "dumped" by his regular physician and elevates psychiatric illness to a respectable position in the patient's mind. This requires that it have a respectable position in the *primary physician's* mind!

No introduction to the field of psychiatry would be complete without a discussion about confidentiality. It's striking how many physicians disregard this important concept. Suffice it to say that the topic of conversation in a psychiatrist's office is usually not the local weather forecast. The physician, privy to important and potentially embarrassing information from his patient, must do everything possible to safeguard his relationship with the patient. Otherwise, the patient will lose trust in his doctor and all hope of getting to the root of his problems will be gone.

Now, you're the psychiatrist, and you're going to be asked to manage a variety of different kinds of patients. Along the way, we hope that you will pick up both good diagnostic skills and an attitude of curiosity and patience for your patient with psychiatric problems.

CHAPTER 2. PSYCHOSES

As a busy psychiatrist, you're asked to come see a "raging, incoherent" man in the emergency room. Armed with your psychiatrist black bag (your brain, a Hold and Treat form, and a pen) you're on your way to stamping out mental illness. The patient is clearly out of touch with reality, nonsensical, and loudly shouting unmentionables, and you must now figure out from what variety of psychosis he suffers. A principle tool in the diagnosis of psychoses is the mental status examination.

There is no way around it, you simply must remember certain fundamental questions that every patient with bizarre behavior or mentation should be asked. The mnemonic, JOIMAT, is provided to help organize your thinking about these patients. Just remember that many acutely psychotic patients wind up in a seclusion room with lots of mats. There isn't much joy in a seclusion room, but at least you can be happy that your patient is not wreaking havoc in other parts of the hospital. Here's a review of quick and simple ways for testing various parts of the mental status examination.

J: *Judgment:* It is important to find out whether the patient can understand acceptable patterns of behavior and consequences of his actions. This can be determined by questions like "If you found a stamped, addressed envelope in the gutter, what should you do with it?" This can help elicit whether the patient understands that such a letter should be put in a mail box. Of course, many of us would pick up the letter and open it to see if there was any money in it. That's why, when you ask the question, you should say, "What *should* you do with it" rather than *would.* In lieu of a formal question, observations about the appropriateness of the patient's behavior can be useful in evaluating judgment.

O: *Orientation:* This refers to whether the patient understands who he is, where he is, and what time it is. Patients should know the day of the week, the date, and the year. Sometimes, disorientation to *time* can be subtle. It may be of value to ask the patient specifically what time of the day it is or even whether he can judge when 60 seconds have elapsed. If the patient is off by more than 15 seconds, suspect disorientation. *Time* disorientation usually accompanies a delirium. Disorientation to *place* is also common in patients with a delirium. Disorientation to *person* is very unusual and seen only in severe CNS dysfunction, amnestic states, and in some patients who are malingering.

I: *Intellectual functioning:* This refers essentially to the patient's cognitive status. How well can he carry out calculations and other thought processes that would be commensurate with his education? Attention span and concentrating ability are also measured by these tasks and are diminished in delirium and dementia (often in depression, too). Ask the patient to subtract 7 from 100, and to subtract 7 from that answer, etc. Trouble subtracting serial 7's occurs in delirium and dementia. With patients who have less than a high school education, try serial 3's from 50. Then ask if he knows the current and past four presidents. If his intellectual capabilities are diminished, this also suggests delirium, dementia or amnestic state.

M: *Memory/mood:* This tests whether the patient can recall both distant and recent events. Examples of distant events are time and place of marriage, assuming the patient is married and not a newly-wed. For short-term memory, the patient is asked to remember three unrelated objects and to recall them five minutes later. Unless the patient is very anxious, he should be able to remember three objects. Immediate memory is tested by asking the patient to recall digits. He should be able to repeat (forwards and backwards) six digits. This is also a test of attention. Describe mood (see Chapter 1).

A: *Appearance/affect:* The patient's appearance (e.g., disheveled, sad faces, motor activity) can be helpful in the evaluation. Disheveled appearance occurs in dementia, moderate to severe depression, and schizophrenia. Increased motor activity accompanies mania. Decreased motor activity occurs in depression. An unusually neat and tidy appearance occurs in obsessive-compulsive states. Describe affect (see Chapter 1).

T: *Thought:* A variety of tests are done in this category. The process of the patient's thinking is important. Do his thoughts relate to each other logically, or do they seem random, having no bearing or relation to each other (e.g., loose associations (see Chapter 1))? What is the content of his thinking? Does he have delusions? Does he have hallucinations? If so, are they visual or auditory? Ask the patient to interpret a proverb (e.g., what does it mean to say "don't count your chickens before the hatch.")? Observe his response. If he answers concretely (e.g., "of course, you can't count chickens until they hatch"), he has lower intelligence or dementia. If his answer is bizarre or idiosyncratic (e.g., "my chickens peek out of the egg, so you can count their beaks"), he probably has schizophrenia. Likewise, a loose answer indicates schizophrenia (e.g., "chickens fly and are hard to count, and my eggs are all in one basket, but the Denver Nuggets won last night."). If he is suspicious and won't answer, he might have paranoia. An answer with clanging associations could indicate mania (e.g., "chickens pop out and poop out, but when they peep out, you can't count them out.") Questions about suicidal ideation should also be asked.

As a rule of thumb, the mental status examination should not be performed at the beginning of an interview with the patient. Some effort should be made to converse with the patient, helping the patient feel that you are there, allied with him in helping him with his problems. But after his mental status examination is performed, you are in a good position to categorize this patient as having a psychosis. Table 1 is provided to help sort this out.

Although the mental status examination is most helpful in diagnosing these various conditions, other information is also of value. Table 2 provides additional data that might be gathered from the patient to help corroborate one of these diagnoses.

Bipolar Disorder (Manic Depressive Illness)

This very curious and common disorder of affect regulation usually begins in the patient's 20's or 30's and involves periodic episodes of either severe mania or se-

TABLE 1

	J	O	I	M	A	T
Schizophrenia	poor	W.N.L.	usually o.k.	memory, o.k. mood, variable	disheveled appearance, flat affect, inappropriate to content of speech.	delusions, hallucinations, paranoia, loose associations
Mania	poor	W.N.L.	may have very good concentration or may have flight of ideas	memory, ok. mood, expansive	affect euphoric, irritable, depressed, flamboyant dress, increased motor activity	grandiose hallucinations, delusions, flight of ideas
Dementia	poor	+/− disoriented to time & place; rarely to person	impaired	memory, impaired mood may be surprisingly without distress	affect may be depressed, labile or inappropriate	+/− paranoia delusions, hallucinations, loose associations, perseverations
Paranoia	o.k. except regarding the delusion	o.k.	o.k.	memory o.k. mood often irritable	affect suspicious appearance o.k.	paranoid delusion, no hallucinations
Delirium	poor usually	disoriented to time and place, rarely to person	impaired	memory impaired often mood variable	affect & appearance variable	may have delusions and/or hallucinations (usually variable)

TABLE 2

	Age of onset	Type Hallucination	Family History
Bipolar Disorder	20-40	Usually Auditory	Usually +
Schizophrenia	15-30	Usually Auditory	Sometimes +
Delirium/Dementia	Any age	Usually Visual	Rarely +

vere depression. Generally, these episodes last from 3-8 months (provided no treatment is implemented) and are interspersed with periods of relatively healthy adult functioning. In fact, many people with manic depressive illness actually function at a hypomanic level (very energetic but not fully in a manic phase) and can get extraordinary amounts of work and chores done. Eventually, though, these patients will enter a manic phase which is characterized by euphoria, pressured speech, extreme motor hyperactivity, hypersexuality, sleeplessness, social intrusiveness, and other impulsive behaviors, often self destructive. When such patients enter a depressive phase, which actually occurs more commonly than the manic phase, the reverse is true. A depressed mood, decreased motor activity, retarded speech, hyposexuality, and sleep disturbance may be the cardinal symptoms (fig. 3).

The *elevated mood* seen in mania can be quite difficult to recognize. Most often, these patients are also irritable. When prevented from doing something that they have their mind set on, they can react with both irritation and angry outbursts. Sometimes lacunae of depressive mood accompany the elevated mood.

Pressured speech, not dissimilar from the speech of someone who has abused amphetamines or recently drunk ten cups of coffee, is characterized by sensical but fast and loud locution. In its extreme form, pressured speech is sometimes termed flight of ideas. Generally, a manic-depressive patient will make sense to an interviewer, whereas a schizophrenic often seems nonsensical. Sometimes the distinction is difficult.

Hyperactivity is a relatively non-specific psychiatric symptom. Motor outlets for feelings are commonly employed by children, but are also seen in anxious and manic-depressive adults. An inability to sit still, constant crossing and re-crossing of the legs, and fidgeting with arms and hands may be the outward manifestation of this aspect of the illness. Sleeplessness is also extremely common.

In addition to these cardinal symptoms, a variety of other problems can accompany manic depressive illness. Typically, the history of these patients reveals that they have been spending money wildly. Although this behavior is characteristic of the housestaff who has recently graduated and entered private practice, it is abnormal when the patient reports having no money or is delusional about how much

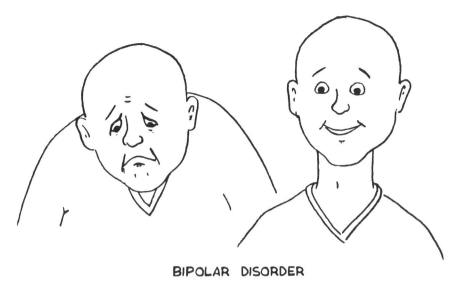

BIPOLAR DISORDER

Fig. 3. Same person, different days.

money he or she has. A loss of touch with reality is almost always present and can be accompanied by frank delusions, usually of a grandiose nature, and hallucinations. Hallucinations are interesting phenomena and can be very useful when trying to distinguish various kinds of organic and functional disorders. Table 3 is provided as an easy reference for the differential diagnosis of hallucinations.

Schizophrenia

No psychiatric disorder is more disabling than schizophrenia. The term schizophrenia has been misused to describe patients with "split personalities." Schizophrenia actually refers to a very specific psychotic illness. Schizophrenic patients

TABLE 3

Hallucinations

	Olfactory	Auditory	Visual	Tactile
Illness	Temporal lobe seizures	Usually Schizophrenia	Delirium	Cocaine abuse (formication)
	Any other	or Bipolar		delirium tremens

are those with chronic thinking disorders (DSM IV): (1) bizarre delusions, (2) paranoid delusions if accompanied by hallucinations, (3) hallucinations, or (4) loosening of associations accompanied by other psychotic symptoms (e.g., catatonia). Although delusions can't be categorized on the basis of the content, in many ways schizophrenic delusions are unique. A feeling that the television is personally communicating with the patient, and the feeling that the patient's thoughts are being controlled by someone else are examples of schizophrenic delusions (fig. 4).

The age of onset of schizophrenia is usually late adolescence to early adulthood. This can be useful diagnostically when the mental status examination is ambiguous. Although the diagnostic findings above are most valid in distinguishing schizophrenia from other psychoses, there are additional diagnostic criteria. Eugen Bleuler coined the term schizophrenia and devised his 4-A's theory at the turn of the century. The 4-A's stand for:

Autism: Idiosyncratic ideas and attitudes. (also see Chapter 1).

Associations: The schizophrenic patient has loose associations (remember Pegasus?).

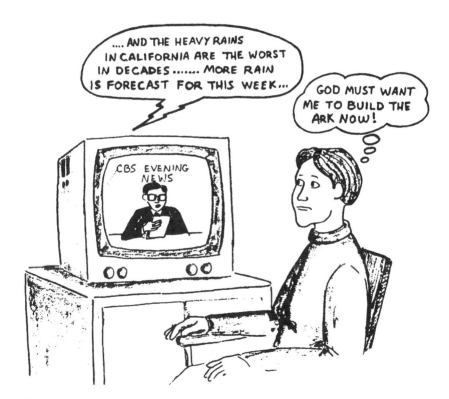

Fig. 4. Idea of reference.

| Ambivalence: | Ambivalence refers to an inability on the patient's part to make up his or her mind. In the extreme, ambivalence may cause paralysis of action; e.g., the patient stands in a doorway for hours, unable to decide whether to enter or leave. |
| Affect: | The affect in schizophrenic patients is typically "flat" (diminished intensity) or inappropriate to the content of their speech. |

An acute schizophrenic decompensation is usually perceived by the patient as frightening and disorganizing. In reaction to a sense of fragility and accompanying paranoia, these patients may become both violent and impulsive. Actually, acute schizophrenia is more accurately referred to as schizophreniform illness because the prognosis is much better when a patient recovers quickly ($<$ 6 months). It's not uncommon for schizophrenic patients to self-medicate (as with sedatives, alcohol, or even amphetamines). Needless to say, this can cloud the diagnostic picture. Chronic schizophrenics often have fixed delusional symptoms which serve as their basic orientation to the world. They may have little apparent anxiety and maintain that they have no problems at all; it's just that the FBI has some special mission for them—that's the problem.

One other aspect of schizophrenia bears mentioning. Catatonia is an accompanying feature in some schizophrenic patients. Catatonia refers to a disorder both of motor control and speech that develops in several conditions. In the schizophrenic, waxy flexibility (patient maintains an enforced posture) and mutism are features of catatonia. Occasionally, agitated catatonia can develop. This type of catatonia is characterized by extreme psychomotor agitation and requires emergency psychiatric intervention, either in the form of rapid tranquilization or ECT. We'll have more to say about these forms of treatment later. Schizophrenia is often classified according to the predominant symptomatology (DSM IV). *Disorganized* schizophrenics have a disorganized behavior, inappropriate or flat affect and looseness of associations. *Paranoid* schizophrenics have predominantly paranoid and grandiose delusions. They also have hallucinations. *Catatonic* schizophrenics suffer catatonia. *Undifferentiated* schizophrenic patients have psychotic symptoms but don't fit any other category.

The risk of suicide is high in schizophrenia, especially in male patients under 30. Depression and suicidal ideation should be evaluated and often requires hospitalization.

Delirium/Dementia

The patient with delirium or dementia may present as clinically psychotic. The principle manifestations of dementia are memory impairment, and other cognitive difficulties. Disorientation to time usually occurs in the early stages of a delirium, and to time, place and, rarely, person in later stages. When a dementia develops gradually, the patient may have time/be able to compensate for his impaired cognitive functioning. When it develops quickly, there is usually acute confusion (delirium), anxiety, and even depression accompanying the disorder. *Perseveration,* repeating of the same words or phrases, also can develop.

As you noticed in the glossary of terms, a delirium is usually considered reversible, and dementia is usually considered irreversible. Delirium develops over a short period of time and may be worse at night. This is termed *sun-downing.* Clouding of consciousness occurs in delirium. Dementia usually develops gradually and affects intellectual abilities.

Delirium and dementia are in fact, symptoms secondary to underlying medical conditions. There are multiple etiologies for these syndromes; therefore, a systematic approach to the patient is necessary to ensure the discovery of the disorder's etiology.

Can a person with an isolated small stroke develop a dementia? Do patients with brain tumors develop the manifestations of delirium? The answer to these questions is usually no. To develop delirium or dementia, the patient must be suffering from CNS disease that affects both cerebral hemispheres. Usually, a stroke affects one area of the brain. If the stroke causes extensive edema, then both hemispheres could be affected. Likewise, a brain tumor won't result in dementia or delirium unless it's very diffuse or very large (large enough to impinge on both cerebral hemispheres). Of course, specific neurologic deficits will accompany punctate lesions in the central nervous system, but memory impairment and disorientation usually occur in the company of diffuse CNS disease. Knowing that, let's explore the types of disorders that can cause these problems.

Endocrine disorders: In the more severe stages of these diseases, endocrine dysfunction affects the entire body, as well as the entire brain. Disorders such as hypothyroidism, Addison's disease, ketoacidosis, and hypoglycemia can cause a delirium.

Drug ingestions: Since drugs are systemically distributed, many drugs can cause a delirium (e.g., ethanol, barbiturates, hallucinogens).

Metabolic conditions: Liver failure, renal failure, heart failure, respiratory failure, and significant serum and electrolyte abnormalities would be expected to affect the entire brain and, therefore, are occasionally responsible for the development of delirium.

Infections: Any infection that involves the entire brain would be expected to cause a delirium. Meningitis and encephalitis occasionally present in this fashion. How about a brain abscess? If you answered that question "yes," then you, too, may be suffering from delirium or dementia. A brain abscess would cause focal neurologic findings; it would cause these disorders only if it were huge, causing swelling or compression of most of the brain.

Intrinsic CNS disease: Large brain tumors, massive strokes, and head trauma do occasionally present as a dementia. More typically, these disorders present in other ways. Arteriosclerotic brain disease is frequently cited as a cause for dementia. However, *only* patients with multiple, small infarcts affecting large areas of the brain would be prone to develop a dementia.

When does a delirium become a dementia and vice versa? There is no easy answer to this question. Some forms of brain insult are irreversible, while others are quite readily reversed. In general, the quicker the diagnosis is made and the faster the underlying medical condition is reversed, the better the prognosis. These syndromes can present at all ages. By the way, a 65 year-old man presenting with acute onset of bizarre delusions and hallucinations would not have schizophrenia, because that illness is never seen developing at this age. As you have noted from the hallucination chart, visual hallucinations are most commonly seen in organic brain syndromes. This is frequently a helpful distinguishing factor.

For teaching purposes, we have simplified the nomenclature for delirium and dementia. The above schema should serve you well in diagnosing most of these conditions, but please remember that exceptions exist: (1) If your patient has had a personality change, but still has intact memory and orientation, suspect a brain disorder. An example of this would be a conservative business man who begins acting radically because he has a frontal lobe tumor. (2) Delusional patients may be suffering from an ingestion, especially of cocaine, amphetamines, caffeine, or hallucinogens. Memory and orientation could be spared in this case, although the cause is substance induced. (3) Selected stroke syndromes and drugs (e.g., amphetamines, reserpine) can cause mood disorders. (4) Hallucinations can be caused by organic conditions. Sometimes memory and orientation are not affected.

Delusional (Paranoid) Disorder

A circumscribed delusion, or delusional system with other mental functioning spared, characterizes delusional disorder. This disorder presents in adulthood and may not come to the psychiatrist's attention. Such patients are often adept at keeping their delusions secret. The DSM IV describes several types of delusional disorder: erotomanic, grandiose, jealous, persecutory, somatic, and unspecified. Acute and chronic forms exist, the latter being more difficult to treat. Paranoia can be a symptom of other illnesses, including schizophrenia, severe depression, organic brain syndromes, and drug ingestions.

A folie-a-deux is an unusual disorder in which two people share the same paranoid delusion. People with *paranoid personality disorders* are extremely suspicious or jealous but do not have delusions.

Now, we return to that wild and agitated patient whom you were called to see at the beginning of this chapter. With your mental status exam and knowledge of the major forms of psychosis, you are able to pin the diagnosis down. Unfortunately, with these kinds of patients, life is usually not so simple as walking into the examining room and taking a careful history. Some of these patients are agitated and combative and would most likely take a swing at you, if you were not careful. Therefore, in conducting your interview and evaluation, it's important to make sure that you, yourself, are safe and that your patient is protected from himself. So, if you have to go see a patient like this, be sure to have a hospital security guard or two accompany you, and be sure not to let the patient head for the hills. We'll have more on the treatment of these disorders later.

CHAPTER 3. THE DEPRESSED AND SUICIDAL PATIENT

Depression develops in fifteen to twenty-five percent of the adult population at some time in life, so you can see that depression is one of the most common illnesses a physician encounters. Unfortunately, many primary care physicians overlook this problem allowing it to remain untreated. The purpose of this chapter is to alert the general physician to the significance and clinical spectrum of depressive illness. Suicide is a frequent concomitant of depression, so we'll be discussing it, too.

Theories about the etiology of depression began with the "black bile" theory of the ancient Greeks which stated that too much bile causes changes in affect. Today's leading theories are somewhat more sophisticated versions of the ancient one. Theories that certain neurotransmitters, particularly norepinephrine and serotonin, are relatively depleted or inactivated in certain areas of the brain in patients with severe depression may seem bilious. However, they offer great promise in understanding the etiology of this illness. Depressed patients often have low levels of metabolites of serotonin and norepinephrine. Also, the fact that depressed patients occasionally have altered dexamethasone suppressing capability (a dose of dexamethasone does not inhibit cortisol secretion the way it normally does), suggests that endocrine factors may play a role in depression.

Attempts at classifying the clinical syndromes or types of depression have met with variable success. Certain dichotomies have been used to describe the ends of the depressive spectrum. For instance, in *psychotic* (as opposed to neurotic) depression, there is a loss of reality testing. *Exogenous* depression occurs in response to an identifiable stress, whereas the cause is not apparent in *endogenous* depression. Depression may be *primary* or *secondary* (some people, for example, get depressed secondary to another illness). *Unipolar* depression is depression alone, whereas *bipolar* depression is depression alternating with mania. Depression may be major or minor. We think that it is most useful clinically to consider depression as occurring along a continuum of mild to severe.

Severe depression may occur anytime in the lifespan and is more common in women than in men. It is termed Major Depression in DSM IV if symptoms are present most of the time, every day for 2 or more weeks.

Let us use the mnemonic, JOIMAT, from the previous chapter and run through a mental status examination in a severely depressed patient.

J: *Judgment* may be impaired, particularly with respect to a patient's view that his situation is hopeless.

O: *Orientation* is usually normal, but in a severely depressed patient, time orientation may be abnormal.

I: *Intellectual functioning* may seem impaired, because attention and concentration are also impaired. Recall that intellectual functioning is also impaired in dementia. It is important to include dementia in the differential diagnosis of depression.

M: *Memory* may appear impaired in depression because depressives have trouble concentrating.

A: *Affect* is, of course, depressed, and often there is a history of crying spells. Extremely depressed patients may have slowed movements and almost blank expressions. This is usually called psychomotor retardation, but if severe enough might be called catatonia!

T: *Thought content* may include ideas of hopelessness or helplessness. Suicidal ideation may or may not be present. Delusional thinking, such as paranoia or believing that the patient's internal organs are rotting, may occur. Behavioral symptoms, also referred to as vegetative signs of depression, are critical to the diagnosis. These include a history of weight loss and decreased appetite, and disturbed sleeping (either difficulty remaining asleep or early morning awakening). Classically, the severely depressed patient awakens at 2-4 a.m. and is unable to return to sleep. Depression and anxiety are often most intense in these early morning hours. The intern gets up at 2 a.m., because his beeper goes off. He has trouble returning to sleep, because he's angry, not because he's depressed. Other behavioral symptoms include decreased sexual interest and slowed motor movements. Constipation is a classic physiological or behavioral symptom of depression.

When the diagnosis is unclear, a personal history of recurrent depression or a family history of depression or manic-depressive illness can help corroborate the diagnosis. Alcoholism in the patient or his relatives can also support the diagnosis. These are risk factors for depressive illness.

It's worth repeating that making this diagnosis is important, because depression is debilitating. Untreated depression usually lasts up to one year. As many as fifteen percent of patients with severe depression may ultimately commit suicide. Despite this, depression is an illness that responds well to appropriate treatment. Ninety to ninety-five percent of depressed patients respond to either antidepressants or electroconvulsive treatments and show a significant remission of symptoms.

At the other end of the spectrum are the mild cases of depression. In mild depressions, judgment, orientation, intellectual functions, and memory are rarely impaired. Thought content may include ideas of self-depreciation or guilt (as in more severe depression), but extreme hopelessness or helplessness and psychotic thinking are not present. Vegetative signs also contrast with severe depression in that weight loss is unusual; weight gain is actually more common. Sleep disturbances occur at sleep onset, and psychomotor retardation is not present. Mild depression is more common in the afternoon and evening hours as opposed to the early morning hours. Constipation is unusual, but diarrhea occasionally occurs. Sexual interest is usually impaired in mild depression, too. Treatment with antidepressants is probably as effective as in severe depressions and patients more often request medications, since the newer drugs have fewer troubling side effects. Psychotherapy is often an appropriate treatment, whether the illness is mild or severe. Dysthymia is the official term for mild to moderate depression which is intermittent over 2 years or more. Dysthymia also responds to antidepressants.

Patients often come to psychiatrists with the simple complaint of "depression." Other frequent presenting symptoms include fatigue, crying spells, difficulty sleeping, and lack of interest in one's usual pursuits. These are the *vegetative signs* of depression. Unfortunately, depressed patients sometimes present symptoms in confusing ways. For example, depressed children might arrive at your office with a complaint of hyperactivity or antisocial behavior. Elderly depressed patients might complain of memory impairment. Somatic complaints (lower back pain) can herald a depressive decompensation.

A number of medical illnesses figure in the differential diagnosis of depression. Among these, hypothyroidism is very common. All patients being evaluated for depression should be asked about other symptoms of hypothyroidism (cold intolerance, hair loss, weight gain).

Cancer of the pancreas frequently causes depression. The reason for this is unknown. Both Addison's disease and Cushing's syndrome can cause depressive features. Certain drugs cause depression (reserpine, alphamethyldopa, propranolol); even viral illness can cause patients to become depressed.

The psychiatric differential diagnosis is equally important.

1. Schizophrenics feel depressed sometimes, especially several weeks to several months after their first decompensation. However, they also suffer from hallucinations, bizarre delusions, and loose associations.

2. Demented patients experience memory impairment and disorientation. Severely depressed patients can appear demented. This syndrome is called *pseudodementia*. Occasionally, dementia has to be diagnosed after a trial of antidepressant therapy has failed.

3. Bipolar patients may be floridly depressed, but also have a history of manic episodes.

4. Normal grief can be very difficult to distinguish from depression. Grief is such a ubiquitous and important response to loss that we will now digress and discuss it.

Grief

Grief follows the perception of a loss. Usually, the loss is a relative or close friend. People will also grieve over the loss of a limb, loss of body functioning, or loss of self-esteem (as in losing a job). Depressed people may develop their illness in the absence of an actual loss; they seem more likely to suffer vegetative signs than those who are bereaved.

There are characteristic stages in grief reactions. People who are grieving experience shock; that is, they initially feel emotionally overwhelmed by their loss. This is usually followed by anger, denial, sadness, and then some form of resolution in which the lost relative, friend, or limb is gradually given up. Grieving typically lasts for about a year.

Pathological grief occurs when grief is intolerable. Watch for these signs to make a diagnosis of pathological grief.

1.   If a surviving relative develops symptoms of the deceased relative, this is a manifestation of pathological grief. For example, a grieving widower whose wife died of colonic cancer might develop stomach aches as a sign of pathological grief.

2.   Suicidal ideation and behavior is also on the pathological scale of grief reactions.

3.   Psychosomatic reactions (ulcerative colitis, rheumatoid arthritis, etc.) and hyperactivity also are aberrant reactions of grief.

4.   Grief lasting longer than 2 years is pathological.

Grieving people do feel depressed and unhappy for a period of time. In the end, the distinction between grief and depression can be difficult. Table 4 summarizes these two clinical states.

Suicide

The evaluation of the suicidal patient is one of the most difficult tasks faced by the psychiatrist. Although fifteen percent of patients who are severely depressed may commit suicide, significant numbers of suicides occur in the absence of depression. The setting of a suicidal act is usually one in which a person experiences intense stress. Such stress leads to affects or feelings which are completely intolerable to the patient. If the person sees no solution to the circumstances causing these intolerable affects, suicide begins to appear as "the only solution" to the situation. This is the time of *suicidal crisis* and can last a few hours to a few days. If assistance is provided, this suicidal crisis can be overcome. The patient's situation may require hospitalization or family support; the priority of this phase of the illness is to safeguard the patient.

TABLE 4

	Depression	Grief
Loss	+/−	+
Thought	guilt, self-deprecation	thoughts of lost relatives/ hallucinations of the deceased relative are sometimes normal. Guilt.
Timing	6–12 mos. +	1–24 mos. following a loss
Depressive Vegetative Signs	Usual	Less Common

A three to nine month period of heightened vulnerability to suicide follows. This post-crisis phase should involve continuous monitoring of the patient. During this phase of the illness, the patient's underlying problems should be treated. For example, if he is depressed, antidepressants are usually indicated. If he has poor coping skills, efforts should be made to teach him new ways of dealing with stress.

The problem during the acute and subacute phases is how to decide the actual risk for suicide attempt. No easy answer exists, but a variety of demographic and psychological data can be elicited to help you decide. Just remember SUICIDAL (fig. 5)!

S: The *Sex* of the patient is important. More men *commit* suicide; more women than men *attempt* suicide. Availability of *Significant* others is also important. Married patients are less likely to commit suicide than single ones, and divorced patients are at higher risk than married ones. The quality of personal relationships is also important. A patient's feelings of loneliness or isolation from important people in his or her life may lead to suicidal thinking.

U: *Unsuccessful,* previous attempts, contrary to popular wisdom, make it more likely that an additional suicide attempt will end in death. An accurate history about previous attempts is crucial. It should include the means previously used (to assess their lethality), the presence or absence of other people at the time(s) of the attempt(s), the patient's distance from medical help at the time(s),

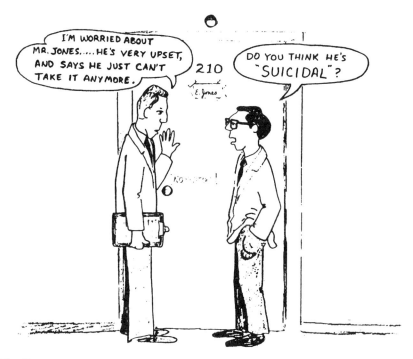

Fig. 5.

the presence or absence of loss of consciousness, and the length of stay(s) in the hospital following the attempt(s).

I: *Identification* with family members who have committed suicide in the past may make suicide a more acceptable option to some patients.

CI: *Chronic Illness,* psychological or medical, and/or recent onset of severe illness is an increased risk factor for completed suicide. Patients with depression, psychosis, and panic disorder are definitely at higher risk.

D: *Depression* significantly increases the risk of suicide as does drug abuse.

A: The *Age* of the patient is important. A simple rule of thumb is that older men are at greater risk for suicide. Young schizophrenic males are at high risk. *Alcohol* use is also common in successful suicides. A patient acutely intoxicated with Alcohol or other substance will be more impulsive and more likely to kill himself. Chronic alcoholism is also a risk factor for suicide. The patient's *Alliance* or therapeutic relationship with the people who are evaluating his suicidal potential should be considered. Patients who are assessed to be most isolated and out of touch with other people are at greatest risk.

L: *Lethality* of suicidal method is an important factor in the assessment. The use of guns, hanging, and jumping from high places are the most lethal means. Greater caution is therefore indicated with these patients. Drug overdoses and wrist cutting are generally less lethal. Recent *Losses* (death, divorce, loss of job) are also critical factors in assessing potentially suicidal patients.

Assessing suicidal potential involves the consideration of many factors. Complicating this assessment is the fact that some patients attempt suicide to manipulate "significant others." Usually, such patients are managed differently than others. It is safer, however, to assume that they are genuinely suicidal at first. If you're certain they are manipulative and don't really want to die, then hospitalization, giving in to the patient's threats, and even psychiatric treatment may not be indicated. These are tough cases, though, and consultation with a psychiatrist or psychiatric colleague is recommended before making these difficult treatment decisions.

Physicians in primary care will see the majority of depressed and suicidal patients. A significant number of patients who commit suicide have seen a doctor in the preceding several months. This suggests that they want help but can't ask for it directly. Remember SUICIDAL and you'll save lives!

(See Chapter 13 for treatment approaches).

CHAPTER 4. THE SLEEPLESS PATIENT

When sleep disorders strike, trouble with daytime functioning or sleeping can develop. Although rarely are sleep disorders life-threatening per se (except sleep apnea), they cause enough distress to warrant careful work-up and treatment. It is useful to identify sleep disorders as being either primary or secondary.

A word or two about sleep physiology is in order. Sleep normally progresses through stages. After four stages have been traversed, REM (rapid eye movement sleep, when people dream) occurs. The deep stages of sleep (3 and 4) predominate early in the night, while REM sleep is more common later in the night. Passing from stage 1 to REM sleep takes about 90 minutes, then back to stage 1, then REM, and so on.

Primary Sleep Disorders

First, let's consider narcolepsy, one of the most unusual conditions. This sleep disorder consists of cataplexy (sudden loss of motor tone when the patient experiences a strong emotion), daytime drowsiness, sleep paralysis (upon awakening, the patient is transiently paralyzed), and hypnogogic hallucinations (hallucinations experienced on falling asleep). Sleeping EEGs (electroencephalograms) demonstrate that REM sleep occurs at sleep onset rather than its usual appearance after stages one to four. These patients need not have all four symptoms.

Treatment consists of amphetamines and tricyclic antidepressants; dosages can vary. These drugs usually suppress the symptoms, thus improving the patient's quality of life.

Dysomnias and parasomnias are discussed in Chapter 10. These are sleep disorders that occur during the deep stages of sleep.

The etiology of sleep apnea can be either central or peripheral. Sleep apnea is a condition of respiratory pause during sleep leading to multiple short arousals, often to hypoxia and hypercarbia ($\uparrow$ pCO_2), and to the sense of having a poor night's sleep. Central sleep apnea is presumed secondary to a problem in the respiratory center of the brain. Peripheral apnea is thought to be caused by anatomical closure of the upper airways, especially the pharynx, during sleep. Occasionally, obesity and hypothyroidism are associated with sleep apnea.

Unfortunate complications can arise with this illness. Hypoxia can cause cardiac arrhythmias and cor pulmonale. Daytime drowsiness can be severe. Treatment can consist of weight loss (which presumably reduces fat tissue in the pharynx), nighttime monitoring, or the daytime use of stimulants. Central nervous system depressants like alcohol and sedative-hypnotics should NOT be used! They aggravate the problem.

Secondary Sleep Disorders

A potpourri of conditions can lead to secondary sleep insomnia. These underlying conditions probably account for most complaints of insomnia. To organize your thinking about secondary insomnia, just remember DEEP. *D*rugs, *E*nvironment, *E*motions, and *P*hysical (medical) problems can cause insomnia.

D: *Drugs*

Understandably, stimulants like caffeine, amphetamines, and decongestants can cause insomnia. They stimulate the central nervous system and can cause sleep problems. Somewhat paradoxically, alcohol and even sedative-hypnotics themselves can cause insomnia. Although alcohol can make the onset of sleep easier, its effects wear off, leading to fitful sleeping later in the sleep cycle. While sedatives induce sleep, they disrupt the sleep cycle if used for prolonged periods (> 2 weeks). Physiologically, they suppress REM and deep sleep. After a few weeks, REM and deep sleep break through, or "rebound" occurs.

Any drug with diuretic action can cause trouble sleeping, because the patient has to get up to void. Beta-blockers (like propranolol), digitalis, antidepressants, pentazocine, and baclofen can cause nightmares. Obviously, a *Drug* history is important in the work-up of insomnia.

E: *Environment*

A surprising number of cases of insomnia are caused by *Environmental* problems (e.g., noise, other stress). A snoring spouse or noisy home could make sleeping difficult (fig. 6). Irregular work shifts or sleeping in a strange bed can cause sleep disruption. Worries about an exam, rendez-vous with future in-laws, or first day of an internship could also transiently disrupt sleep.

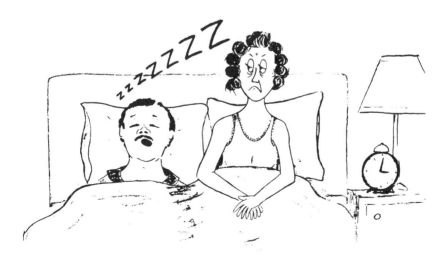

Fig. 6. The Environment is noisy.

E: *Emotional*

While worrying sometimes causes a fitful night's rest, more severe psychiatric illnesses cause profound sleep disruption. Mild depression causes trouble falling asleep, and severe depression results in early morning awakening. Mania causes so much agitation that sleeping is almost impossible. More severe anxiety states consistently affect sleep patterns. Schizophrenia probably does not specifically affect sleep, but it does cause agitation and anxiety, which will affect sleep. Delirium usually causes gross disruption of the sleep-wake cycle. Paranoid people may not be willing to let their guard down long enough to sleep. The above disorders are discussed at length in their respective chapters.

P: *Physical problems*

Anyone in *Pain* is going to have trouble falling asleep. It's harder to stay distracted at bedtime than during the day, and distraction keeps one's mind off pain. The antidepressant, amitriptyline, often helps sleep disturbance caused by chronic pain and may decrease pain as well.

Likewise, medical illnesses, particularly those which require hospitalization, can cause sleeping problems. Certain medical conditions actually strike at night or during sleep (paroxysmal nocturnal dyspnea secondary to heart failure, nocturnal angina). Short-term usage of hypnotic drugs may be indicated, as long as the drugs don't aggravate the underlying condition.

The differential diagnosis of sleep trouble is relatively simple. A sleep lab can help firm-up a diagnosis by running a sleeping EEG on your patient. You'll help a lot of people, if you can get them to sleep. Just remember DEEP!

CHAPTER 5. THE ANXIOUS PATIENT

Most physicians don't respond to a request for an antianxiety medication by reaching for their prescription pads, but a systematic approach to the problem of anxiety is a difficult task. Anxiety is a prominent symptom in many psychiatric and medical disorders. Anxiety also accompanies frightening or distressing situations. For example, examinations arouse anxiety! We would like to provide you with a method to systematically approach the problem of anxiety, so you won't be nervous the next time an anxious patient enters your office.

Anxiety cannot be quantified. It's a subjective symptom comprised of the moods of apprehension and worry. It also has physiological components of motor tension and autonomic hyperactivity. Anxiety occurs either "spontaneously" (primarily), secondary to other psychiatric conditions, or secondary to medical disease. For the sake of this discussion, we'll consider anxiety about the National Boards (or other strong stimuli) to be normal (whew!), unless the anxiety results in avoidance behavior. If you skip the test, or if your hand is shaking so hard that you can't write answers to the questions, that's a problem.

Deciding what constitutes normal versus pathological anxiety can be difficult. Let the patient tell you how distressed he feels. His subjective experience is important. Look for behavioral changes designed to avoid anxiety, such as staying at home all day instead of going to work. Your subjective impression of normal and abnormal behavior is also important. Try to judge whether the anxiety is appropriate to the situation.

Be aware, too, that patients may not complain of anxiety per se. Complaints of light-headedness, tingling in extremities, hyperventilation, and a sense of "unreality" are often expressions of anxiety.

Primary Anxiety Disorders

Primary anxiety conditions include phobias, panic attacks, generalized anxiety, post-traumatic stress disorders, obsessive-compulsive disorders, and dissociative episodes. Fifteen to twenty-five percent of the population will develop an anxiety disorder in their lifetime.

Phobias are illogical fears of situations, animals, places, and so on. They typically are single or isolated (only one phobia per customer) and are appreciated by the patient as being illogical. Desensitization therapy—gradually increasing the exposure of the patient to the feared situation—usually successfully treats phobias.

Panic attacks occur out of the clear blue and result in transient, acute, severe anxiety. Patients with this condition eventually get anxious about becoming anxious and begin to do things to try to avoid panic (e.g., staying in the house all of the time). For unclear reasons, several benzodiazepines, tricyclic antidepressants, fluoxetine, other selective serotonin reuptake inhibitors, and MAO inhibitors

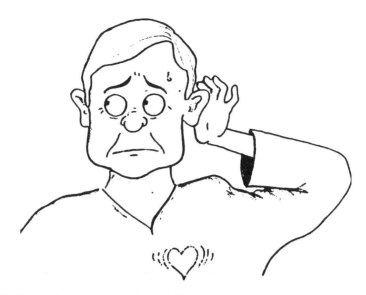

Fig. 7. Generalized anxiety. He's vigilant.

work in this condition. Now, patients suffering from panic attacks have a good chance of quick recovery.

Some people are anxious all of the time. They manifest a sort of hypervigilance and autonomic hyper-arousal. These people, who suffer from *generalized anxiety,* would be likely to complain of increased sweating, palpitations, apprehension, the feeling that "something" bad might happen, or anxiety. The cause is unknown, but psychotherapy with or without antianxiety medication is treatment of choice (fig. 7).

When a person has been exposed to a severe stress (e.g., being physically or sexually abused as a child or adult, seeing a relative murdered, serving in Viet Nam), he may be anxious and upset for years. Events that remind him of his traumatic experience (like a TV show about murder) might trigger anxiety, bad dreams, aggressive outbursts, or flashbacks. The treatment for this disorder is psychotherapy aimed at helping the patient integrate his past traumatic experiences. Antianxiety and antidepressant medications are also occasionally helpful.

Obsessive-compulsive traits describe anxious people who try to squelch their anxiety by thinking or performing rituals. Obsessive-compulsive traits are common in many people, especially physicians. Such traits are normal unless the physician feels he must check his doctor's orders form a hundred times before leaving the hospital. In that case he has *obsessive-compulsive* disorder. Effective treatment can consist of psychotherapy, behavioral modification, or medication. Clomipramine is a new drug on the U.S. market for obsessive compulsive disorder. Fluoxetine, a new antidepressant is also effective for this problem.

Dissociative episodes are experiences in which the patient feels his mind is separated from body. These are often seen in post traumatic stress disorder, occur in clusters, occasionally brought on by strong emotions, and can be treated with psychotherapy and/or antianxiety medications. Seizures sometimes present as dissociative episodes and should be considered in the differential diagnosis.

Anxiety Secondary to Psychiatric Disease

Certain psychiatric conditions are notorious for generating high amounts of anxiety. First, and foremost, is schizophrenia. The feeling of losing one's mind, hearing voices, or having delusions is extremely frightening. Antipsychotic medications are not specifically antianxiety, but they do help dampen the distress.

When demented people realize that their memory is failing, they may suffer what is called a catastrophic reaction. Enormous amounts of anxiety and panic accompany the utter incomprehension associated with this illness. Anxiety can accompany delirium, too.

Thirty to forty percent of depressives suffer anxiety.

Anxiety Secondary to Medical Conditions

Some medical conditions cause anxiety and should figure in the differential diagnosis. Consequently, a history should be taken and a physical exam done on anyone whose chief complaint is nervousness. As a general rule, the anxiety secondary to a medical condition can present like any of the psychiatric manifestations of anxiety (e.g., dissociative episodes, generalized anxiety, panic attacks, etc.)

First, consider the possibility that a drug(s) is causing the problem. Anticholinergic properties can cause anxiety (antipsychotics, tricyclics, etc.). Nicotine, amphetamines, cocaine, and coffee can cause anxiety. Sedative-hypnotics occasionally induce paradoxical arousal and anxiety. Alcohol and sedative-hypnotic withdrawals typically cause restlessness, anxiety, and elevated vital signs. Hallucinogens can cause anxiety, because the perceptual changes they induce may be frightening.

If no drugs are involved, move on to common medical problems. Hyperthyroidism can cause agitation and anxiety. Hypoglycemia can induce anxiety symptoms, because it causes secretion of epinephrine. Cardiac arrhythmias occasionally cause nervousness. Surprisingly, mitral valve prolapse is frequently associated with panic disorder. Hypoxia also makes people nervous and agitated.

Still no luck? Then it's time to consider the rare birds (fig. 8). Pheochromocytomas secrete catecholamines, which cause intermittent symptoms of anxiety. Acute intermittent porphyria, insulinomas (by causing hypoglycemia), carcinoid tumors, and even temporal lobe epilepsy have been implicated in anxiety symptoms.

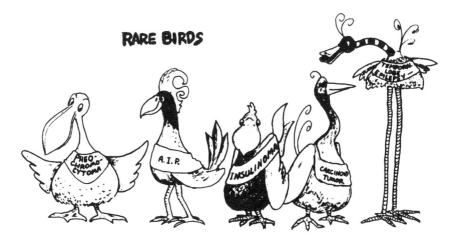

Fig. 8.

Finally, don't forget that anyone who is ill may feel nervous about the illness. Although this should be considered normal situational anxiety, it may be an indication for treatment. For example, patients immediately after myocardial infarction may need antianxiety treatment to help prevent the development of arrhythmias. Agitated, anxious patients may need medication if they are in traction, need to be still, or are suffering significant psychological distress.

CHAPTER 6. PAIN

Although the differential diagnosis of pain includes a wide variety of psychiatric and physical ailments, the experience of pain is valid no matter what the underlying diagnosis. Remember this and you'll be off to a good start with patients who complain of pain. Eventually you'll form the kind of relationship with them that will alleviate the pain. That's right! When a patient believes he is being well cared for, he'll feel less pain. This is true whatever the etiology of the pain.

Before discussing the differential diagnosis of pain, we would like to say a few words about placebo treatments. Placebos are often used as a way of "proving" that the patient is not in pain. Such misuse of placebos often damages the doctor-patient relationship. A patient's response to a placebo only indicates that the patient is a placebo responder. It does not mean that the patient has no pain. Most likely there are physiological mechanisms that are triggered in response to the suggestion that something will relieve pain. These underlying physiological mechanisms actually relieve pain and probably involve endorphin-mediated pain relief. Endorphins are endogenous opioids. If a patient is a placebo responder—and this should be diagnosed only with the patient's permission in advance—then the patient may be able to get by with decreased dosages of pain relievers. In other words, it's great to be a placebo responder! Again, the power of suggestion and a relationship of trust are critical to good patient management.

A complaint of pain, with no identifiable physical reason for the patient to have pain, indicates the psychiatric differential diagnosis. The remainder of this chapter will discuss this diagnostic category and give you clues and advice on managing such problems. This information is summarized below in table 5.

Depression

Why does the heading "Depression" appear in a chapter on pain? Have these guys lost their minds? Surprisingly, depression may be the most common cause of pain. Pain can function as a depressive equivalent—a ticket of admission—to the physician's office. Lower back pain, headaches, vague chest pains, and aching extremities may all be presenting complaints for depression.

The diagnosis of depression is covered in depth in Chapter 3. Remember, even when patients complain of something other than a depressed mood, it is often possible to diagnose the depressed mood. Simply ask the patient how he or she is feeling and look for other signs of depression. Does the patient appear sad or apathetic? Look for the vegetative signs of depression (anorexia, constipation, sleep disturbance, weight loss, decreased libido). If you suspect depression, a trial of psychotherapy or tricyclic antidepressants is indicated.

TABLE 5

	Psychological Findings	Affective State	Pain Distribution
Depression	vegetative signs, hopeless, helpless	depressed	lower back pain typical
Hypochondriasis	strong need to be cared for	anxious	internal organ or varying complaints
Malingering	history of trouble with law, or substance abuse	neutral or angry	story inconsistencies
Munchausen's	needs to fool doctors	anxious and demanding	abdominal pain
Conversion	the symptom symbolizes something	indifferent or anxious	loss of neurologic functioning often does not follow anatomical pathways

Hypochondriasis

A hypochondriac is someone who believes he has a serious medical illness despite medical assurance to the contrary. Hypochondriacs frequent clinics and private offices in search of someone who will take care of them. Their wish is often frustrated, because many doctors pat the patient on the back, tell him that nothing is wrong, and send him out. If this happens, the patient goes to another doctor's office. The law of averages states that you will occasionally obtain a prescription from a doctor no matter what your complaint. Consequently, these patients wind up with a list of prescriptions that reads like a hospital formulary.

This condition can be difficult to diagnose. Hopefully, if you've shown concern for your patient, he'll come back to you rather than doctor shopping. Hypochondriasis is suggested when the same person visits your office 4 5 times a month with complaints that are unmatched by physical disease. A patient's use of 15 medications that seem unnecessary also can be a clue to this diagnosis. If you feel annoyed with these patients at times, you're in good company. This type of patient frequently arouses countertransference feelings in doctors. Countertransference refers to feelings doctors have for their patients. This countertransference can diagnose a hypochondriac. Of course, if you are annoyed all day long with all of your patients, it isn't countertransference! It's probably the car trouble you're having, the argument you're having with your spouse, or low Board score that you just made (fig. 9).

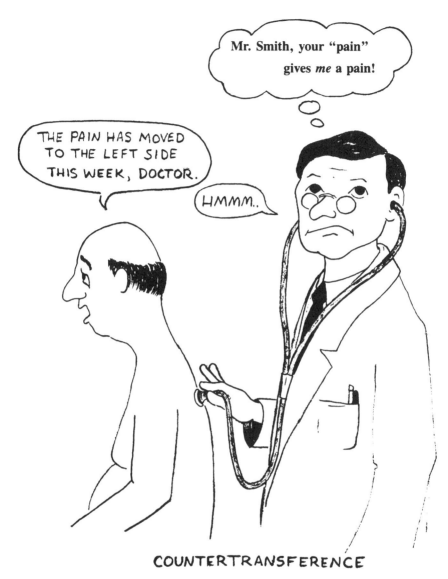

COUNTERTRANSFERENCE

Fig. 9.

The best way to manage the hypochondriac is to treat him or her with under-standing care. In other words, take his complaints seriously, listen carefully to his history, tell him that you are worried about him, and see him regularly, albeit briefly. You don't have to give him any medications (unless something is war-ranted); you also don't have to be a psychiatrist to treat this person. It's surprising how helpful you can be by showing your concern for your patients. Inevitably, a hypochondriac occasionally develops a "real" illness, too. That's all the more reason for taking his complaints seriously.

You also shouldn't feel obliged to treat these patients. A full case load of hypochondriacs is undesirable. Some people have trouble managing these kinds of patients and should refer them.

Conversion Disorder

Conversion disorder usually refers to a loss of voluntary nervous function without any identifiable physical pathology. Pain without any underlying neurologic problem can also be a conversion disorder. Conversion disorders are uncommon these days. The classical hemipareses, fainting episodes, and hysterical (conversion) seizures of yesteryear just aren't seen as much in the 1980's. Instead, conversion symptoms are more subtle. Vague pain, transient visual disturbances, or transient motor weakness can be conversion symptoms.

The conversion symptom symbolizes the patient's wish to do something and the defense against that wish. For example, a concert pianist could develop numbness and tingling in his fingers for conversion reasons. He can't play the piano because of his symptoms, which functions as a defense against the wish to play piano, or be famous.

The differential diagnosis for conversion disorder is extremely important. More than twenty percent of those diagnosed as having a conversion disorder are found subsequently to have true organic pathology. The psychiatrist and neurologist must be humble when they can't find a reason for the patient's initial loss of motor or sensory functioning. Aside from conversion disorder and the other psychiatric conditions that can cause pain, several neurologic disorders can present like a conversion disorder. Multiple sclerosis often presents with vague neurologic symptoms. The diagnosis of M.S. is based on the development of multiple C.N.S. lesions over a period of time. Laboratory confirmation is often possible in the diagnosis of M.S. Acute intermittent porphyria, Wilson's disease (altered copper metabolism), and small infarcts also may cause symptoms that appear to be conversions, but these are obviously organic problems.

Corroborating psychological data can help lead you to the diagnosis of a conversion disorder. First, conversion patients may appear mildly indifferent to the loss of some significant motor or sensory functioning. This classical "belle indifference" is not unlike denial, though. Please don't place too much importance on this symptom.

If a patient has had previous somatic complaints or conversion symptoms, it's more likely that the current loss is for conversion reasons. If a family member has had a similar neurologic loss, your patient most likely has a conversion symptom, and is identifying with his relative's symptoms. Patients who are the youngest sibling are more prone to have conversion symptoms. A loss of motor or sensory functioning that follows an immediate psychological stressor is more often due to a conversion disorder than a general medical problem.

Unfortunately, conversion disorders can co-habitate with neurologic conditions. Patients with multiple sclerosis, true seizures, and head trauma seem to be at higher risk for developing conversion symptoms. This obviously adds to the confusion.

The treatment of a conversion symptom starts with an honest discussion with a patient. Statements such as "I'm sorry we don't have an answer, but we think both the psychiatrist and the neurologist should follow you" keep the patient involved in both neurologic and psychiatric care. Hopefully, later, the diagnosis will become more obvious. Ultimately, the psychiatric treatment of such patients tries to uncover the symbolism behind the loss of functioning. When a medical student is allowed to discuss how much he wants to slug his resident, his right arm's paralysis may improve. The longer the conversion symptom lasts, the worse the prognosis. Consequently, a patient with a conversion symptom of three years duration is less likely to benefit from psychiatric treatment.

Malingering

Here is the one exception to the rule to take a patient's complaint of pain seriously. Some patients will come to your office or hospital, complaining of pain, in order to get narcotics or a hospital bed to sleep in. In other words, they aren't actually in pain. They are consciously trying to persuade you to give them something. While some malingerers are drug abusers, many are impoverished patients who have nowhere to spend the night. Although you don't take their complaint of pain seriously, you can still treat them empathically (and also emphatically!).

A diagnosis of malingering should be suspected when the patient does not have any psychological concomitants of the other pain conditions. If the patient has a history of drug abuse, malingering should be suspected. A patient who has been in trouble with the law isn't likely to have many qualms about being dishonest with you, either.

Treat such patients firmly but compassionately. Occasionally, referral to a social service agency will be helpful (to help the patient find a bed for the night, etc.) Often, though, these patients will leave the hospital when they are denied drugs or a hospital bed. Sometimes, these patients are dangerous. If you suspect that the patient you are seeing might try to hurt you, call for help in the form of guards or orderlies. If you have access to a psychiatrist, he or she can help you diagnose malingering and make an appropriate disposition.

Factitious Disorder (Munchausen's Syndrome)

Patients with Factitious Disorder consciously want to fool their doctor, but they don't know *why*. These are patients who show up in the emergency room with "gridiron" abdomens and with histories of multiple prior surgeries with nothing ever discovered. Their symptoms and complaints are convincing.

Suspect this diagnosis if a patient has a history of multiple surgeries with no reasons (i.e., tumor, disease); if the patient has received medical treatment in many different cities; if the patient is a transient and doesn't have much in the way of family support. Generally, there is not history of drug abuse or other obvious psychopathology. The best management for this condition is psychiatric consultation. Factitious Disorder by proxy is a type of child abuse whereby a parent induces an illness in his or her child in order to fool the doctor. Examples include injecting toxins into a child or giving a child medicine to make him sick. Invariably the parent is medically trained.

The treatment of pain should follow several principles. To reiterate, proving that a patient is a placebo responder does not prove that he is pain-free. Secondly, when a patient has acute pathology (e.g., status post abdominal surgery), there is no harm in giving him good pain relief with narcotics. Withholding needed pain meds can obviously produce demanding, drug seeking behavior which, when finally reinforced by the provision of medication, can become a major source of conflict for staff and patient. There is almost no chance of turning a medically or surgically hospitalized patient into a narcotics addict provided narcotics are only dispensed when the patient experiences pain.

When patients are distracted by a good television show or family visit, they will subjectively experience less pain. Obviously, keeping patients involved in activities is therefore one way to obtain non-narcotic pain control. In the unlikely event that a patient does develop a physiological dependence on narcotics, the withdrawal syndrome for narcotics is generally not life-threatening. Narcotics withdrawal is similar to a flu-like condition and poses few medical problems in its management.

CHAPTER 7. EATING DISORDERS

Although we'll crack a few jokes in this chapter about eating disorders, there is nothing funny about a person suffering from anorexia nervosa or bulimia. These illnesses, particularly anorexia nervosa, can be *devastating*. Psychological anguish experienced by such children and adults is severe; the frustration experienced by families is often extreme.

To make this subject more palatable, we've arranged the diagnostic findings for anorexia nervosa into an acronym, LOW FORM. The diagnostic findings in anorexia nervosa are:

L: *Loss*
O: *Of*
W: *Weight:* There is a weight loss in excess of 15% of ideal body weight.
F: *Fear of*
O: *Obesity:* These girls are terrified about being fat.
R: *Refusal* to eat occurs despite family and medical intervention.
M: *Miscellaneous* symptoms include the following, most of which are secondary to weight loss: amenorrhea, lanugo hair growth, bradycardia, vomiting and purging, and laxative abuse. One symptom, body image disturbance, is manifested by the belief of these girls that they are overweight despite actually being emaciated (fig. 10).

Please look for LOW FORM in anyone who has lost weight. Remember, not every thin child has anorexia nervosa. A variety of medical problems can mimic this psychiatric condition and should not be overlooked. We'll have more to say about the differential diagnosis later.

The epidemiology of anorexia nervosa is interesting and worth knowing a little bit about. The incidence of this disorder is on the increase, probably due to social and cultural factors. Thin is beautiful in the U.S.A. One in 200 girls at puberty is now thought to have anorexia nervosa. The disorder is much more common in girls than in boys, and it occurs more commonly in Jewish and Italian families. Middle and upper class families are at greater risk for having a child with this disease than are lower socioeconomic status families. The most common age of onset is the teenage years, the illness may be preceded by a period of mild obesity and mild dieting. There is also an association of anorexia nervosa with Turner's syndrome and with above-average intelligence.

No one knows the cause of this disease. Theories about the development of the disorder can be divided into three categories. The traditional psychoanalytic model assumes that anorexic patients have a deep fear of sexuality and of impregnation. These fears are accompanied by the fantasy that impregnation occurs via the oral route. That's why these patients stop eating, because they don't want to get pregnant! Although this theory is hard to stomach, it does make sense for some of these patients. The second, more palatable theory, is one of endocrinologic dysfunction. There are endocrine abnormalities in anorexia nervosa (including increased vaso-

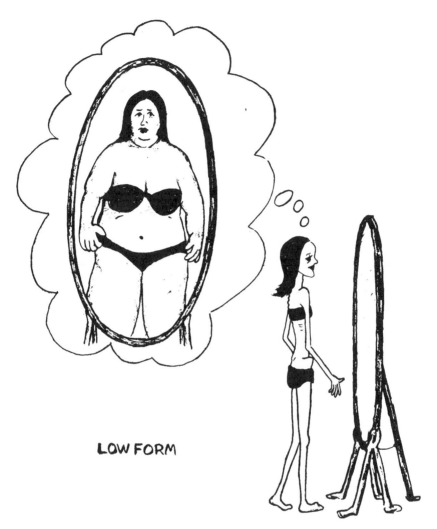

LOW FORM

Fig. 10. Anorexia Nervosa.

pressin levels and alterations in thyroid function). These may reflect some underlying endocrinological etiology. Girls who develop amenorrhea often do so prior to any significant weight loss. This also suggests that an endocrine imbalance causes this disorder. A third theory for the etiology of this condition could be termed an interactional model. Early in childhood there are interactions between parent and child that could lead to a child refusing to eat at an older age. For example, an impatient mother could habitually rush her daughter through meals. This pressure could make it difficult for the girl to enjoy eating. She probably would develop a wish to control her own eating pace. At an older age she might actually refuse to eat.

By now, you are becoming familiar with the diseases in the psychiatric differential diagnosis for anorexia nervosa. Obviously, a schizophrenic patient could be delusional about food. He might think that he was being poisoned, and would understandably stop eating. The resulting weight loss could be misperceived as anorexia nervosa. Remember to look for LOW FORM. Bulimia involves binge eating followed by some form of purging (including vomiting or increased exercise to atone for overeating) in patients who otherwise maintain their weight. An important aspect of bulimia is that gross overeating is followed by excessive guilt. Depressed patients lose weight, also. They should describe feeling depressed, other vegetative signs of depression (remember JOIMAT), and even suicidal ideation. They also don't suffer from LOW FORM.

On the medical side of the differential diagnosis are a variety of conditions that should be considered. Addison's disease can present with weight loss, anorexia, and vomiting; electrolyte abnormalities should indicate the diagnosis. Hypothyroidism may present with cold intolerance, constipation, bradycardia, and skin changes that are similar to those seen in anorexia nervosa. However, hypothyroid patients are often overweight and should have other physical stigmata of this disorder. Other chronic illnesses can cause progressive weight loss, but these should be readily discernible (i.e., inflammatory diseases, chronic infection, and malignancy). Any disorder that causes panhypopituitarism could initially mimic anorexia nervosa. The superior mesenteric artery syndrome sometimes causes vomiting and anorexia. The vomiting usually occurs when the patient is lying down, though. Diabetes insipidus (DI) causes excess fluid intake, but behavior and attitudes related to solid food are usually normal. Recent research shows that some schizophrenic patients have D.I. Any patient with D.I. should have a medical work-up and mental status examination!

Psychiatric patients with LOW FORM can get into medical difficulty. Five to fifteen percent of anorexic patients die, usually of fluid and electrolyte difficulties. Always check the electrolytes, vital signs, EKG, and mental status of your patient. Why check the mental status when you already have LOW FORM? A small percentage of these patients have recurrent suicidal ideation.

After you have ascertained that your patient is medically stable, the treatment commences. Usually, an inpatient psychiatric facility will be required to prevent the patient from continuing to diet. Certainly, there is no problem with an outpatient trial of psychotherapy if the patient is not in medical difficulty. You should be aware of things that anorexia nervosa patients do to themselves. A small percentage of them abuse laxatives; a greater percentage self-induce vomiting. Most of these patients distort the amount they are actually eating. This is not done from real maliciousness, but because they are desperate not to gain weight. So, when your anorexia nervosa patient appears at the nurse's desk in the morning with a big smile on her face, two pounds heavier than she was the day before, be suspicious! She may have put metal in her pockets, ingested three gallons of water, or put batteries in her shoes. Of course, you may be doing such a superb job, that she has actually gained weight, too. She probably wouldn't be smiling in that instance.

The treatment of these girls should consist of behavioral modification to reinforce *weight gain,* and some combination of individual and family psychotherapy. When a patient's weight drops to a critical point, she should be forced to eat. If she refuses, a nasogastric tube or intravenous hyperalimentation becomes mandatory. It is usually possible to prevent a patient with anorexia nervosa from dying from complications of the disease. A variety of interventions can be made to prevent starvation.

The prognosis is guarded in anorexia nervosa, with many patients never fully recovering from their obsessional concern with weight. Some patients may go on to develop full-blown affective disorders (depression); a few make a full recovery.

Before moving to the next section, we pose one puzzler. Why do so many anorexia nervosa girls appear orange? Is it some odd liver failure syndrome that accompanies starvation? No! It's hypercarotenemia, caused by the ingestion of too many carrots and raw vegetables.

While anorexia nervosa patients may both gain and lose weight, another class of patients gain and never lose—obese patients. This may be the least understood of all psychiatric conditions. Certainly the cure rate for severe obesity (100% heavier than ideal weight) is low.

A reasonable approach to understanding and working up obesity is to use a differential diagnosis. First, obesity can be caused by medical problems. Probably, fewer than five percent of obese patients have an underlying medical condition. It doesn't hurt to consider hypothyroidism, Cushing's disease, Prader-Willi Syndrome (hypothalamic dysfunction) and side effects of antidepressant and antipsychotic medications and lithium as possible etiologic conditions.

Having ruled these out, move onto the secondary obesity syndromes; i.e., those that are secondary to an underlying psychiatric condition. Obsessional eaters, depressives, anxious people, and even schizophrenics can suffer from obesity because of their underlying condition. The treatment here should be aimed at the underlying problem.

Last, not least, but least understood are the primary obesity syndromes. We list a few hypotheses for why some people become obese.

1)   Some patients, fearful of "looking good," choose (unconsciously or consciously) to stay obese so they won't have to deal with intimate relationships or sexuality.

2)   Some obese people learn to deal with their frustration or anxiety (beginning at an early age) by eating. They substitute oral gratification for other kinds of gratification.

3)   An undiscovered problem with sense of satiety could exist (mmmm!).

4)   The set point for eating and weight gain could be set too high in some people, implying that we all tend to stay at approximately the same weight unless this set point changes.

One thing is certain, psychiatrists don't have much luck using conventional treatments with these people. A psychiatric evaluation may be indicated to rule out other psychiatric conditions, but psychotherapy doesn't usually help. Amphetamines have anorexic properties but aren't safe to use for this condition. Increased risk of medical complications (coronary artery disease, hypertension) is true, especially for the severely obese, but doesn't usually affect the patient's behavior, either.

Psychiatrists are relying more on behavior modification (reinforcing weight loss), nutritional counseling, and their other medical colleagues! In severe obesity, the only effective treatment may be surgery (ileo-jeujunal by-pass) or supervised calories restriction.

In moderate obesity (20% heavier than ideal weight) calorie restriction and behavioral modification to encourage weight loss are probably most effective. In mild obesity, no treatment or moderate exercise and calorie restriction may be indicated. Not all obese patients want treatment, and obesity is not synonymous with psychopathology.

Pica is a condition in which people eat non-food substance items (paint chips, dirt, wood, etc.). Iron deficiency can cause pica; many children eat unusual items accidentally or out of curiosity.

Although the presence of pica can imply that a child is not being adequately cared for, the side-effects of eating odd items are more serious. Lead-based paint chips can cause lead poisoning. Any child with pica should have his or her home environment carefully checked.

CHAPTER 8. ALCOHOL AND DRUG ABUSE

Alcoholism

Alcohol use is common and usually poses no medical or psychological problems. Alcohol abuse is a major public health problem. You may have heard the rumor that alcoholism has replaced syphilis in Osler's famous phrase, "He who knows (this disease) knows medicine." Here's why.

Between five and ten percent of the population suffers from alcoholism (defined below). This equals ten to twenty million Americans. A significant number of patients hospitalized in general medical hospitals have alcohol related problems. Cirrhosis of the liver, a problem frequently associated with alcohol abuse, is the eighth leading cause of death in the USA. In some areas, fifty percent of homicide victims are legally intoxicated; twenty percent or more of suicide victims are legally intoxicated; at least fifty percent of fatal automobile accidents are associated with alcohol abuse.

Even such diverse accidental causes of death as burns, carbon monoxide poisoning, and private plane crashes are frequently associated with alcohol abuse in the victims. So-called "accidents" are the fourth leading cause of death overall and the number one cause of death in both men and women up to age 34. The incidence of alcohol abuse is high among accident victims!

Alcoholism affects all socioeconomic groups but men more than women. Per capita consumption of alcohol is on the increase.

It's as hard to define "alcoholism" as it is to recognize it. When a person drinks so much that it interferes repeatedly with adequate adult functioning (socially, occupationally), this should be considered alcoholism. Some people can drink a lot and still get by, but if they develop tolerance to alcohol (need to drink more to get same physiological effect), this, too, should be considered alcoholism. When a person has withdrawal symptoms after stopping drinking (see below), he should be considered an alcoholic. Although vulnerability to the end organ affects of alcohol consumption varies, when end organ disease is present, suspect alcoholism. The occurrence of blackouts (memory loss during periods of intoxication) also suggests alcoholism (fig. 11).

Alcohol ingestion without chronic abuse can lead to problems, too, including pathological intoxication (one or more drinks causing a major personality change), acute intoxication, coma, and death.

Many factors are thought etiologic in the development of alcoholism. Patients with a family history of alcoholism have been shown to be more likely to develop alcoholism in adult life. Cultural influences are also extremely important. In some cultures, alcohol use is frowned upon but intoxication is implicitly accepted. In other cultures, alcohol use is the norm but intoxication is unacceptable. The availability of alcohol also leads to its use. This obviously is an important issue in setting age limits on alcohol use. Some personality traits seem to be associated with alcoholism, particularly antisocial and borderline personality disorders.

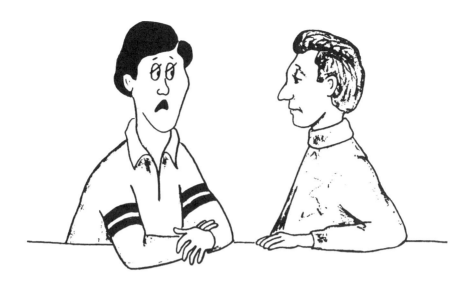

IT SOUNDS LIKE I HAD A TERRIFIC TIME
LAST NIGHT....... WHAT DID I DO AFTER
I CLIMBED THE FLAGPOLE?

Fig. 11.

Before discussing the treatment of alcoholism, let's run through the myriad complications of alcohol abuse. First are the "medical" complications. Gastrointestinal disease (peptic ulcer, gastritis), liver disease (hepatitis, alcoholic fatty liver, cirrhosis and its attendant problems), pancreatitis, cardiomyopathy, anemia, myopathy, and hypoglycemia are all complications of alcoholism.

The neurologic complications include peripheral neuropathy, dementia, cerebellar degeneration, subdural hematomas, and Wernicke-Korsakoff syndrome. This last problem is a life-threatening illness caused by thiamine deficiency that alcoholics can develop. It includes confusion and apathy, ataxia, and abnormal eye movements. If treatment is not instituted (thiamine, 50-100mg I.M. qd × 3), this illness progresses to the irreversible Korsakoff's dementia (confabulation—making up facts—and severe memory impairment).

Alcohol withdrawal syndromes can also be life-threatening. *As a general principle, all sedatives (including alcohol) can cause severe withdrawal problems.* Here are the problems with alcohol withdrawal.

(1) Alcohol withdrawal consists of sweating, elevated vital signs, tremor, *mild* confusion, and discomfort. It starts 8 to 12 hours following the last drink and then lasts up to 48 hours. It is NOT life-threatening. Some discomfort can continue for days.

(2) Delirium tremens (D.T.'s) is a life-threatening withdrawal state that consists of hyperpyrexia and *delirium.* The mortality rate is 10-15%. This syndrome develops later (between 50 and 100 hrs. after last drink) and lasts up to ten days.

(3) Withdrawal seizures develop 12-36 hours following the last drink. Remember that a variety of other problems could cause seizures in an alcoholic, including infection, head trauma and metabolic problems.

(4) *Alcoholic hallucinosis* consists of hallucinations developing in a patient with an otherwise normal mental status examination.

The psychiatric complications of alcoholism may be the worst. Loss of friends and family, job, and self-esteem can all accompany alcohol abuse. Dementia is the end product of prolonged abuse. Depression and abuse of other drugs are also associated with alcoholism.

Alcohol treatment has several components, which can be divided into *withdrawal management, rehabilitation,* and *follow-up with support.* In most cases, a request for treatment of alcoholism is precipitated by a threatened loss. The doctor may think that the patient has come for treatment voluntarily, but a threatened loss such as that of a loved one, a job, or personal freedom (as in going to jail for alcohol-related legal problems) is often found when a careful history is taken. Also, an obstacle to successful alcohol treatment is the patient's denial of his drinking problem. Denial in an alcoholic may manifest as frank lying, refusing to admit to problems despite great contradictory evidence, or blaming others for his problems.

Alcohol withdrawal can be accomplished on either an inpatient or outpatient basis, depending on severity of withdrawal symptoms. Medical problems should be stabilized, good nutrition implemented, and pharmacotherapy implemented, if necessary (e.g., chlordiazepoxide, clonidine and others to help quell withdrawal signs and symptoms).

The rehabilitation phase of alcoholism treatment is variable in length. This phase of treatment may be accomplished on an inpatient or outpatient basis. When the patient has a previous history of D.T.'s, very bad impulse control (frequent fights, spending binges), a history of seizures, or major underlying psychiatric problems the treatment should begin inpatient. Essential components of treatment include education about the physiological and psychological effects of alcohol, including how the patient's alcoholism affects his relatives, employer, etc. Treatment also aims to help the alcoholic find a way to replace alcohol in his life. Group therapy (see Chapter 11), individual therapy, and self-help programs like Alcoholics Anonymous (AA) can help in this regard.

Low self-esteem is an important psychological issue for most alcoholics, and treatment must address this problem. If the patient is very depressed (and has low self-esteem because of this), his depression should be treated. If he lacks assertiveness and self-confidence, then assertiveness training (in Chapter 11) may be indicated. Group and individual psychotherapy can be of use, too.

The last phase of treatment consists of *support*. Most experts in the field believe that the only reasonable goal for an alcoholic is to completely abstain from drinking. A minority view is that controlled drinking is possible, particularly for those patients who don't have a long history of alcohol abuse or who have not developed tolerance to its effects. To support the alcoholic, AA, family, friends, business, psychiatrist, or a combination of the above can be used. Allowing an alcoholic to become socially isolated courts relapse. Abstinence from drinking may be facilitated for several months by using disulfiram (Antabuse), which interacts adversely with alcohol (see Chapter 11). Abstinence may also be aided by the use of naltrexone (ReVia) and opioid receptor antagonist that has been shown to reduce alcohol craving and thus help to prevent relapse. Self-esteem should continue to be monitored, particularly as it might be affected by continued bouts with alcohol abuse. In other words, relapses occur and should not be treated with admonitions and severe criticism, lest the patient's low self-esteem creep any lower.

Non-alcohol Substance Abuse

Abuse of other substances also poses health problems. We will provide brief clinical descriptions of the effects of a variety of substances that are abused.

Narcotics (heroin, morphine, codeine, etc.) produce physical and psychological dependence. Therefore they cause a withdrawal syndrome if they have been abused for a prolonged time. Availability and cultural factors, again, lead to abuse. For instance, in Viet Nam, where heroin was more readily available and acceptable than in the USA, it was used more. The servicemen who abused heroin in Viet Nam usually did not continue to abuse this drug in America. People who use heroin in the USA probably have more personality problems (extreme dependence, antisocial qualities) than people who don't use it.

Heroin intoxication causes drowsiness, respiratory depression, a sort of euphoria, pain relief, nausea, vomiting, and pupil constriction. Too much of a narcotic can cause coma and death.

Narcotic withdrawal, again, is similar to a flu-like syndrome and *IS NOT LIFE-THREATENING* (unless the person has underlying severe medical problems). Symptoms of "gooseflesh," lacrimation, yawning, mild fever, and irritability can last up to a week. The length of withdrawal symptoms varies directly with the duration of action of the narcotic used.

Treatment consists of a drug program that provides the patient with support, an alternative to the narcotic (methadone, or new relationships), and a new "culture": i.e., new peers who don't support drug abuse or antisocial behavior.

Sedatives (benzodiazepines, barbiturates, methaqualone) have the potential for psychological and physical addiction. *Withdrawal from these drugs can be life-threatening* and usually should be initiated on an inpatient unit.

Hallucinogens (e.g., LSD, psilocybin, mescaline) cause illusions (misperceiving actual sensory stimuli), hallucinations, affective changes, and sometimes panic! Treat acute intoxication with a quiet room and a "talking down" (lots of reassurance). These drugs may have anticholinergic properties, too. Anticholinergic drugs can cause dry mouth, constipation, dilated pupils, hyperthermia, tachycardia, and delirium.

Marijuana use is widespread in America today. This drug (psycho-active ingredient is tetrahydrocannabinol) may not always be harmless. Its acute effects include sedation and a sense of timelessness. A few people who use marijuana will experience paranoia while on the drug and some will have panic attacks. Rarely, marijuana can induce a transient psychosis lasting several hours to several days after its use. Long-term use can cause chronic bronchitis and probably lung cancer. Habitual use can probably lead to an "unmotivated" syndrome. This is a specific attitude toward life that is the result, not the cause, of marijuana use. The drug is not physically addictive.

Marijuana has promising therapeutic effects. It can reduce nausea and vomiting secondary to cancer chemotherapy. It may also have a beneficial effect on glaucoma, but is effective for only a short time, after which tolerance develops.

Cocaine use was more common in middle and upper socioeconomic groups until the last decade. This anaesthetic produces a feeling of euphoria and optimism, making it particularly psychologically appealing. It is physically addictive. The method of usage probably does correlate with whether an habitual pattern of use develops. Intranasal use (snorting) is less likely than smoking ("crack") or IV use to lead to psychological addiction. Common, transient side-effects of cocaine are impaired judgment, elevated vital signs (cocaine has sympathomimetic properties), and grandiosity. Uncommon side-effects are transient psychosis (lasting as long as several days after use), hyperthermia, seizures, and circulatory collapse.

Habitual cocaine use is hard to treat. Successful programs probably have to be coercive to succeed (e.g., threaten to turn you into your employer if you have traces of cocaine in your body.)

In some cocaine users, drug usage takes priority over family and job. Therefore, family counseling may help a family cope with its affected member.

Amphetamines are used for their stimulating and arousing properties. Common side effects include euphoria, anorexia, dry mouth, and elevated vital signs. Uncommon side effects are motor movements, seizures, and circulatory collapse. Psychiatrists are especially interested in one particular side effect. Some users develop a transient paranoid psychosis (lasting hours to several weeks) that can be indistinguishable from paranoid schizophrenia. The drug dosage at which this occurs varies with the individual. Chronic abuse of amphetamines causes tolerance; withdrawal from amphetamines can cause depression.

A variety of other drugs fall in and out of vogue, including paint and glue sniffing, phencyclidine (PCP) abuse, and abuse of combinations of drugs. If you have a high index of suspicion when you examine your patients for liver problems, gastritis, etc., and if you are firmly but empathically confrontive when you suspect abuse, you'll help a lot of patients. Also, please remember that *sedative withdrawal can be serious!*

CHAPTER 9. MEDICAL PROBLEMS
PRESENTING AS PSYCHIATRIC SYNDROMES

In the opinion of these authors, most patients with a psychological complaint should have a careful history and physical examination. The history should look for details of medication usage, age of onset of the mental changes, length, type and duration of the mental status changes, and quality of physical complaints. The physical examination should include a routine physical examination and a careful neurologic examination. The latter is most likely to reveal helpful information in a patient with an abnormal mental state.

A variety of disorders can cause delirium or dementia (see Chapter 2). This chapter will describe conditions that affect the central nervous system. However, the focus will be on diseases that parade as psychiatric syndromes. It will be your job to rain on the parade of these dysfunctions (fig. 12).

A mnemonic to help you categorize these conditions is MED'CL. Unfortunately, there will be some hard work in learning the manifestations of these disorders.

M: Metal poisoning
E: Endocrine
D: Drugs
C: Cancer
L: Lots of others

M: Metal poisoning

Lead intoxication can cause intellectual impairment that progresses to delirium and coma. In chronic exposure to lead, the intellectual deficits can be subtle. In massive or acute intoxication, delirium and coma almost always occur.

Lead intoxication should be suspected in a child who behaves abnormally, especially if he lives in an old house where lead-based paint has been used. Children are more vulnerable than adults to C.N.S. effects. They may become hyperactive, aggressive or irritable after lead exposure.

In adults, the symptoms are abdominal pain, neuropathy and anemia. When poisoning is severe, it may present with neurologic changes (dizziness, ataxia, seizures), lead lines (especially in children, at gingival margins), basophilic stippling in the red blood cells, and optic atrophy.

The treatment consists of supportive measures and chelation treatment to help the patient excrete the lead. Early intervention may not prevent permanent C.N.S. damage, so the best treatment is preventive (e.g., use of unleaded paint, gasoline).

Mercury poisoning causes personality changes. The personality changes characteristically are increased timidity, withdrawal, easy embarrassment, and irritability. The physical changes associated with mercury poisoning include stomatitis, possible kidney and lung disease, insomnia, fatigue and even hallucinations. The neurologic changes are ataxia and tremor. The treatment is a chelator such as

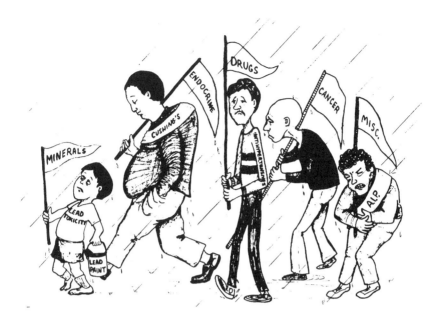

Fig. 12.

penicillamine to help the patient excrete the metal. The personality and neurologic changes are irreversible if the poisoning is severe.

Toxicity develops in people who work in industry involving mercury; e.g., vacuum pump, thermometer manufacturing.

Aluminum poisoning develops after industrial exposure or in chronic renal failure patients. Renal failure can cause hyperphosphatemia. One treatment for hyperphosphatemia has been aluminum-containing antacids. Absorption of aluminum (in the antacid) through the G-I tract can cause aluminum poisoning.

The mental status changes consists of a speech disorder followed by progressive dementia. Eventually, aluminum poisoning causes coma and death. Other systemic changes are osteodystrophy and myoclonus. The best treatment is prevention by monitoring aluminum intake (both orally and in the dialysate).

Manganese intoxication occurs occasionally in people who manufacture batteries. Mental status changes initially are limited to irritability; with chronic manganese poisoning, emotional lability, impulsiveness, and even periodic aggressiveness can develop. Manganese can cause lesions of the basal ganglia, and may cause extrapyramidal signs and symptoms on physical examination. Such patients may also have masked facies and a loss of equilibrium. Unfortunately, there is no treatment for manganese poisoning at this time.

Arsenic poisoning, of course, can cause death in an acute overdose. However, chronic arsenic poisoning is likely to cause the gradual onset of symptoms of inflamed mucous membranes and a dermatitis. Mental status changes would mainly consist of increased lethargy and withdrawal. Severe, chronic arsenic poisoning leads to encephalopathy with marked diminution in intellectual functioning.

Arsenic is found in rodenticides, insecticides, movies, and novels. The treatment is the chelating agent, B.A.L. (dimercaprol).

Bromides, found in old-time medicinal preparations, can cause syndromes that closely resemble psychiatric illness. For example, delirium and schizophrenia-like illnesses have been reported with bromide ingestions. Hallucinations can occur in the company of an otherwise normal mental status exam.

Neurologic symptoms can occur, too, including ataxia, sluggish pupils, and tremor. The treatment is supportive.

Why so much time and energy on conditions that are so uncommon? Two reasons. First, as you can see, these heavy metals can mimic psychiatric illness. Second, you're in a good position to one-up your attending or resident, now.

E: *Endocrine Disorders*

Cushing's disease can present with a variety of mental status changes. The patient may describe feeling moody with periods of euphoria alternating with periods of depression. Occasionally, a patient with Cushing's disease will present with a delirium. By the way, patients on exogenous steroids are at risk for developing these symptoms, too.

The physical changes in Cushing's disease should be familiar to you. There is a movement of fat centrally so that a buffalo hump and obesity develop. Bones may become brittle, and the patient may become hypertensive. Diabetes can develop. The mental status changes can precede the physical stigmata of Cushing's disease.

Addison's disease can present as withdrawal, apathy, and depression. Addison's disease can cause weight loss and vomiting, so it can parade as anorexia nervosa. However, Addison's disease occurs at all ages, has the same incidence in men as women, and does not cause orange discoloration. Patients with Addison's disease are weak, have electrolyte abnormalities, and may have increased pigmentation if the condition is chronic.

Hyperthyroidism also can cause mental status changes, or changes in the patient's behavior. Patients so afflicted can develop hyperactivity, pressured speech, and a type of "mania." They may also suffer from increased irritability and impulsiveness. Obviously, most patients with hyperthyroidism are thin, have elevated vital signs, and have the biochemical changes associated with hyperthyroidism; i.e., abnormal thyroid function tests, e.g. increased T_4 or decreased TSH.

Hypothyroidism will cause depression in some patients. In addition, chronic hypothyroidism can cause withdrawal, apathy, and lack of interest in previously enjoyed activities. Such patients have wasting of the lateral margins of their eyebrows, obesity, diminished basal metabolic rate that sometimes causes depressed vital signs, occasionally signs of myxedema, and "thick tongues." The deep tendon reflexes will be slowed (especially the return phase), helping establish this diagnosis. By the way, please do not start somebody who is depressed on thyroxine. This treatment is ineffective for depression except for the short term and can cause problems for the patient. Too much thyroxine may rev up his system and throw him into heart failure. If he has panhypopituitarism, it can cause him to have an Addisonian crisis. Thyroxine is not a psychotropic medication! (T_3 however is occasionally used to augment the partial response to an antidepressant.)

Hypoglycemia causes anxiety progressing to all kinds of neurologic symptoms, ataxia, and coma. Along the way, personality changes, or a schizophrenia-like illness can develop.

D: *Drugs*

Certain prescription drugs are notorious for causing psychiatric syndromes in patients. The antihypertensives will often cause patients to feel depressed. Reserpine is most likely to do this, but patients on alpha-methyldopa (Aldomet) and propranolol (Inderal) may report feeling depressed, also. Generally, if a patient reports to you a history of major depressions, or if a patient is a "type A" business man, propranolol may not be a good choice of medication to treat his/her hypertension.

Cimetidine, now widely prescribed for the treatment of peptic ulcer disease, can cause a toxic psychosis. As an aside, what's another possible cause of an altered mental status in your patient in the intensive care unit with a bleeding ulcer? Answer: Acute severe blood loss could cause poor perfusion to the brain, resulting in delirium.

Any drug with anticholinergic properties can cause delirium (e.g., tricyclic antidepressants, over the counter sleeping pills, anti-Parkinsonian drugs, antipsychotics). Why does the octagenerian getting an eye examination become confused and combative? Answer: Somebody used eye drops with anticholinergic properties to dilate his pupils. Why does he become confused and combative when his eyes are patched following cataract surgery? Answer: Some patients, particularly the elderly, have marginally compensated mental functioning. When they lose a major source of incoming stimulation (e.g., vision), they can suffer a "mental decompensation." Other eye medications also cause psychiatric symptoms. Their use may be overlooked in the history. Beta blockers (timolol, betaxolol) used to treat glaucoma undergo systemic absorption and may cause depression. Acetozalamide causes anorexia, lethargy, or depression in as many as 40% of users.

Steroids can affect mental functioning in several ways. Some patients develop delirium. Others develop affective disorders (depression or mania). These mental status changes are usually seen with high doses of steroids (e.g., 40 mg/day or more of prednisone).

C: *Cancer*

Malignancies also can cause subtle and not so subtle mental status changes. Pancreatic carcinomas frequently cause severe depression and this can be the presenting complaint. Certain tumors are known to have remote effects on the central nervous system. Lung carcinomas can cause a progressive dementia as well as other neurologic signs and symptoms. Pheochromocytomas can cause patients to suffer from anxiety attacks and "manic" episodes.

L: *Lots of others*

We've saved a potpourri of disorders for last, but not because they're the least important. These are the ones that haunt psychiatrists the most. We'll run through these in list fashion, too. Sorry, there is no easy way of memorizing these, either.

Wilson's disease is a disorder of copper metabolism. It causes pathology in the eyes (Kayser-Fleischer rings), kidneys, brain, and liver. In the brain, it affects the basal ganglia, causing flapping or wing-beat tremors. Most importantly for this discussion, Wilson's disease can cause protean psychiatric complaints. Some patients appear to have nothing short of a classical psychoneurosis. Actually a number of such patients have been psychoanalyzed prior to the discovery of their disordered copper metabolism. Other patients develop a frank psychosis, making it easier to suspect Wilson's disease. The mental status changes usually develop in mid to late adolescence. The treatment is chelation and is usually effective.

Acute intermittent porphyria is a disorder of prophyrin metabolism. AIP usually manifests with abdominal pain, transient neurologic symptoms, and mental status changes. The mental status changes in this disease, too, are protean. Some such patients feel vaguely anxious or depressed, while others appear floridly psychotic. Anyone who has recently ingested a barbiturate who develops these symptoms has AIP until proven otherwise. But AIP can present in other situations, such as times of menses, stress, and other drug ingestions.

Huntington's chorea is a hereditary disease of the brain that usually presents with choreiform movements. An autosomal dominant, it typically presents in the third or fourth decade. Of interest here is the fact that Huntington's chorea can present as a schizophrenia-like psychosis. Sometimes this occasional presentation precedes the onset of the neurologic symptoms and complaints. Ultimately, these patients suffer from a severe and debilitating dementia. What's the diagnosis in a 32-year-old man with "schizophrenia" and tardive dyskinesia (involuntary movement disorder, often secondary to antipsychotic medications)? Answer: Probably schizophrenia and tardive dyskinesia, but be sure to take a careful family history for Huntington's chorea.

Vitamin B12 deficiency can present with a myriad of behavioral changes, including visual hallucinations, personality changes, or a dementia. The history might be positive for a Bilroth procedure and no supplemental vitamins, or chronic, severe malnutrition. Neurologic signs may include weakness, numbness, and tingling of the extremities, loss of proprioception (ability to sense the direction of joint movement), and overactive reflexes.

Pellagra is caused by nicotinic acid deficiency and can be associated with insomnia and delusions. In addition to these mental status changes, the patient would most likely also have a rash, abdominal complaints, and cerebellar ataxia. The four D's of pellagra are diarrhea, dermatitis, dementia, and . . . death if untreated.

Temporal lobe epilepsy is one of the greatest paraders. Although patients with temporal lobe seizures usually have simple automatisms or repetitive behaviors, they may also have schizophrenia-like or manic-like psychoses. When the diagnosis is suspected, an EEG is a sleep deprived state using nasopharyngeal leads should be done. If the diagnosis is still suspected, but the EEG is normal, a trial of the anticonvulsant, carbamazepine (Tegretol), may be indicated. If your manic-depressive patient gets better on carbamazepine, he still could have a psychiatric illness. Some manic-depressives improve on this drug, which suggests that there may be some overlap between mania and temporal lobe epilepsy.

Hypercalcemia can cause almost any imaginable psychiatric symptom, as can *hypocalcemia.*

Hyponatremia can cause weakness, lethargy, and ultimately an organic psychosis (delirium with serious loss of reality testing).

Hypokalemia causes weakness, anxiety, and depression.

Please don't be overwhelmed. Almost all of these disorders will be discovered if you perform a history, and physical examination. Now it's time to go rain on the parade!

CHAPTER 10. PSYCHIATRIC CONDITIONS OF CHILDHOOD

The psychological complaints and symptoms of children can be confusing. Children can be very symptomatic despite no serious psychological problems. Ninety-five percent of children will develop a phobia. Thirty to forty percent suffer night terrors. Enuresis occurs in ten percent of 5 year old boys. When do these and other problems warrant a work-up and/or treatment? This chapter will help you decipher the odd array of symptoms and complaints that children present to their pediatricians, family doctors, and psychiatrists.

Here are some principles of human development. They are provided to help you decide whether the cause of a child's symptom is serious.

1) Generally, chronic exposure to stress in childhood leads to psychopathology. In contrast, exposure to an isolated traumatic event (e.g., one automobile accident, one surgical procedure) usually does not cause lasting personality changes. Some families react pathologically to a traumatic event for their child. They treat the child differently than before. This can cause difficulty for the child.

2) Some development in childhood occurs sequentially and inalterably. For example, it's not possible to walk before you can sit. A child's struggle for autonomy (age 2) precedes his entry into the Oedipal period (age 3-6).

3) Boys are more vulnerable to the development of psychopathology than girls; all childhood disorders are more common in boys with the exception of thumbsucking and anorexia nervosa.

4) Certain traumatic events in childhood will be reactivated throughout the lifespan. For example, a 3-year-old who loses a parent could become seriously depressed or anxious later in life in response to minor losses or separations (such as attending summer camp).

5) Certain psychological symptoms are normal if they occur at the appropriate developmental phase. For example, it's normal for a 2-year-old to be oppositional. Oppositional behavior in a 9-year-old is not normal.

When a child presents with a behavior problem, the history can be important, too:

1) Is the problem chronic or acute? Long-standing problems usually are serious.

2) Is there a family history for psychiatric disorders? Many conditions can be transmitted genetically (e.g., schizophrenia, bipolar disorder, enuresis, alcoholism).

3) How is the child being raised? Is discipline too severe?

4)   Does either parent have a psychiatric disturbance? Children of depressed mothers are more likely to suffer developmental delays than children of "normal" mothers.

5)   Is the behavior problem very disruptive (e.g., fighting in school)? This usually indicates a more serious problem.

6)   Is there a history of divorce? Divorce adversely affects pre-school age children more than older children. Chronic marital discord is probably harder on a child than divorce.*

Now let's move on to the most common childhood problems.

Enuresis

Enuresis refers to wetting at a point in a child's development when he or she is physiologically capable of controlling his or her bladder. Maturation occurs at variable rates in children. That means that a 4-year-old could have occasional loss of control of his bladder and still be within the range of normal. A 2½ -year-old, physiologically capable of bladder control, could have enuresis.

It may be helpful to distinguish between primary and secondary enuresis. The former refers to wetting that has occurred continually in the child's life. The latter refers to enuresis that has developed after a period of at least a year during which the child was adequately bladder trained. *Nocturnal* enuresis is bedwetting that occurs during sleep, usually during sleep stages 3 and 4. *Diurnal* enuresis is either daytime or both daytime and nighttime enuresis. This dichotomy is important, because diurnal enuresis is more likely due to physical problems. Nocturnal enuresis is an example of a parasomnia. Parasomnias are described later in this chapter.

What do you do for a child who has enuresis? Of course, you CAP'IM. You must discover the etiology of the enuresis, always remembering that the vast majority of enuresis is caused by psychological factors.

C: Central nervous system problems can cause wetting, including frontal lobe tumors and spina bifida occulta.

A: Anatomical derangements such as posterior urethral valves can lead to enuresis.

P: The *p*sychological causes of enuresis are varied and are described below.

I: *I*nfections of the urinary tract may result in enuresis.

M: *M*etabolic conditions like juvenile onset diabetes mellitus and sickle cell trait and anemia also can cause enuresis. The work-up is a simple one and should consist only of a careful history and urinalysis unless the history or exam suggests disorders requiring further evaluation. Always avoid invasive procedures unless absolutely indicated, because these procedures cause children psychological trauma.

*Rutter, M. Parent-child separation: psychological effects on the children. *J. Child Psychol. Psychiatry*. 1971; 12:233–60.

Enuresis is a symptom that is self-limited. Psychological causes are varied and include repressed anger, deep-seated ambition, and unconscious difficulties on the parts of other family members expressed in the child's symptom. For example, a father who hated school could subtly encourage his child to wet his pants at school. The symptom is often treated with bladder training exercises or antidepressants, but the treatment should also be aimed at the underlying psychological or medical condition.

Childhood Psychoses

Although debate persists about the nomenclature for childhood psychoses, we think it is clinically useful to divide the psychoses of childhood into two categories. Childhood Pervasive Developmental Disorder (PDD) and symbiotic psychosis.

PDD (DSM-IV) is a disorder that usually commences early in infancy and consists of abnormal language development, abnormal responses on the part of the child to his or her environment, and abnormal social development. The language abnormalities can include echolalia (the child repeats verbatim what he has heard), mutism, pronoun reversals (e.g., the child uses "we" or "you" instead of "I"), and language delays. Typical responses to the environment include a pathological need for sameness. Such children, for example, might become anxious if the furniture in their classroom were rearranged. Their social development is delayed or absent. They show very little interest in other people and are usually found to have delayed or aberrant social milestones in their developmental histories. For example, such children might demonstrate no social outreach, very little smiling, and no interest in the communications of their parents. A descriptive term for this condition is autism.

Obviously, this is a devastating illness. It occurs evenly across all social strata and may be slightly more common in boys than in girls. The disorder can be mimicked by central nervous system damage. For example, congenital infections (rubella, cytomegalovirus, etc.), hepatic encephalopathy, and even massive head trauma could result in a clinical picture indistinguishable from PDD. Children who are congenitally blind have a greater chance of having autistic mannerisms than other children. Complex genetic patterns of inheritance may exist in this condition. Rett's syndrome consists of autistic behaviors plus acquired microcephaly and stereotyped hand movements.

What is clear is that PDD should no longer be considered simply a psychological disorder. These children have abnormal auditory evoked responses, decreased nystagmus in response to vestibular stimulation, and an increased frequency of grand mal seizures prior to adolescence. This suggests that there are organic difficulties that are present in this condition.

The prognosis is not good but varies according to how much language development is present in the child and what his or her IQ is, if this can be tested adequately. The higher the IQ, the better the language, the better the prognosis is.

Treatment should consist of a structured educational program that includes behavioral modification that encourages social and language behaviors. Thioridazine (Mellari) can be useful when severe anxiety is present, but does not affect the underlying psychosis. Recent reports suggest that haloperidol (Haldol) may be helpful in this condition. Psychotherapy for the family can be useful when the family is having a difficult time dealing with the child or when social and environmental factors are thought to be important in the development of the disorder in a particular child.

Symbiotic psychosis is an odd disorder that manifests itself between the ages of 16 months and 30 months of life. In some mother/child dyads or units, difficulty develops on the part of the mother in distinguishing herself from her child. At a time when children are interested in separating from their mothers, this can cause great difficulty for these mothers who have so-called blurred personal boundaries. That sounds complicated, so let's explain with a case.

A typical presentation for symbiotic psychosis would be excessive distress on separation from mother (or father). This distress would abate when the parent was brought back to close proximity to the child. A careful psychiatric evaluation should reveal that the mother can't tell herself apart from her child. For example, one mother recently started herself on a diet, because she thought she was overweight. As she thought that she and her two-year-old son were one and the same, she felt it only natural that she should start her boy on a diet as well. Unfortunately, the child was already thin and began to suffer from failure to thrive, a condition in early childhood in which children don't grow adequately. His presentation in the emergency room was of inanition secondary to his mother not feeding him properly.

The prognosis in this disorder is quite good provided interventions can be made on behalf of the child. A partial parentectomy is indicated to help the child separate from his or her mother. By this we mean gradually increasing the length of time that the child spends away from his/her mother. These parents should be watched closely, because they occasionally have a psychiatric decompensation of their own when faced with the thought or actuality of a separation from their child.

Night Terrors and Other Parasomnias

Parasomnia is a sleep disorder that occurs in the deep stages of sleep (stages 3 and 4). Roughly one third of children younger than five will experience one night terror (Pavor Nocturnis). A night terror is an awakening in the deep stages of sleep accompanied by loud screaming and frenetic behavior. The child's scream may be so blood curdling as to strike panic in the rest of the family, but the condition is normally very benign and self-limited. Occasionally, night terrors are precipitated by daytime stress. For that reason, a cursory history should be taken about these children to make sure that they are not being abused, experiencing inordinate stress, or having other difficulties. Night terrors can be distinguished from nightmares fairly easily. Nightmares have a dream associated with them, occur later in the sleep cycle because they occur with REM sleep, and usually occur in a child who can be wakened without great difficulty.

Sleep talking (somniloquy) occurs during all stages of sleep. It's nothing to worry about, but also can be precipitated by daytime stress.

Contrary to what we see in popular cartoons in which a character gracefully and aimlessly walks a tightrope while sleepwalking, this disorder in children (somnambulism) occasionally is dangerous. Children are not graced with acrobatic skill, and can trip and fall and hurt themselves. A child who sleepwalks should have his room secured, so that there is nothing dangerous to walk into. Otherwise, this condition is fairly benign. It, too, can be triggered by daytime stress.

Childhood Antisocial Behavior

Violent behavior can develop in children. This section will not deal with nomenclatures for childhood aggressive behavior, but will help you to recognize childhood misconduct and to make a referral when appropriate.

Although it's difficult to call a seven-year-old a sociopath, the matrix for adult antisocial behavior is in childhood. No one develops aggressive or antisocial behavior in a vacuum. Exposure to repeated violence at home teaches children that this is an acceptable mode of behavior. When a child who has broken the law or hurt someone is brought to your attention, you should look for the following details in the family history. Look for the VACUUM (fig. 13).

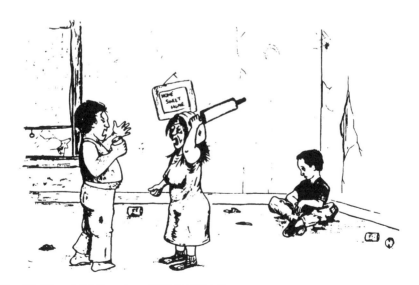

Fig. 13. The child lives in a "VACUUM."

V: *Violence* is often present in the family of a child who has committed an antisocial act (e.g., hurt someone, shoplifted, etc.).

A: *Alcoholism* is more common in families with children who exhibit antisocial behavior.

C: *Child abuse* is frequently found in the family.

U: *Unempathic parenting* can be hard to delineate, but often leads to antisocial behavior.

U: *Underpriviledged class* of itself does not cause antisocial behavior. However, children can learn violent behavior from their environment as well as from their family.

M: *Maternal deprivation* also may predispose to antisocial behavior. Generally, inadequately cared for children grow up feeling angry about this. Their anger can be vented in a variety of areas, including antisocial acts.

If the child has committed a serious crime, the behavior should *always* be taken seriously. If the child consistently breaks minor rules and regulations, this behavior should also be taken seriously. If the child has only one minor infraction and does not live in a VACUUM, you should send the child home without psychiatric treatment. If he lives in a VACUUM and is breaking the law, he's in trouble.

Childhood Depression

Children are not immune from affective disorders. We would like to believe that children grow up happy, but this is not always the case. They can exhibit the same kinds of depressive features as their adult counterparts, with a few noteworthy exceptions.

Children are more likely to develop "depressive equivalents." They may be hyperactive, slightly antisocial, abuse drugs, or fight with their family as a way of expressing an inner feeling of sadness. Usually, the child can report the subjective feeling of sadness or depression.

A special variant of depression can occur in infancy. *Anaclitic depression* occurs in children between the ages of 7 months and about 24 months of life. During this phase of development, children know enough to be able to recognize when their parents are missing, but have not achieved object constancy. That means that when their parents are out of sight, they seem to have vanished permanently. Consequently, children of this age may be affected by separations of lengthy duration (greater than 2-3 weeks) and feel a loss. Depression in infancy looks like depression in adulthood, and is very devastating. For that reason, when children are separated from their parents, as when they become ill and have to be hospitalized, every effort should be made to allow liberal visitations by the parents, or to provide the child with a surrogate nurturing figure (e.g., foster grandparent).

Hyperactivity

Terminology is changing here, also. What used to be called MBD (minimal brain dysfunction) is now termed "Attention-Deficit Hyperactivity Disorder" in the DSM IV. The name has been changed because there is no proof that minimal brain dysfunction causes short attention span. A short attention span can occur with and without hyperactivity. Since hyperactivity is such a common presenting complaint, let's focus on it.

Hyperactivity should be considered a symptom with its own differential diagnosis. This differential diagnosis includes:

Depression: As a depressive equivalent, some children appear hyperactive.

Adjustment reaction: Children who are experiencing anxiety or transient stress may appear hyperactive.

Central nervous system disease: Major central nervous system pathology can cause hyperactivity (e.g., massive head trauma). Minor CNS disease probably does not cause hyperactivity.

Endowment: Some children seem to have a constitutional disposition to be hyperactive. They are described as having had a hyperactive temperament as infants.

Drugs: Sedative-hypnotics can cause a paradoxical reaction in children, resulting in hyperactive behavior. Paradoxical reactions are uncommon in adults. Phenobarbital, commonly used for seizures, may cause some children to become hyperactive.

Vulnerable Child Syndrome: Some parents feel that their children are vulnerable or on the verge of dying. Usually, these children have been very ill previously but have completely recovered. Nevertheless, their parents continue to see them as sickly. They may present as hyperactive. The hyperactivity is a reaction to parental overprotectiveness.

As with any other symptom, the underlying disorder should be treated. Hyperactivity severe enough to interfere with the child's functioning, either at school or at home, may require a trial of methylphenidate (Ritalin), pemoline (Cylert) or other medications. Remember that all medications have side effects; use them carefully.

Tic Disorders

That's *tic*, not *tick*. A tic is a repetitive, purposeless movement. Eye blinking and facial grimacing are examples. Again, boys are more vulnerable. Tics are usually transient (last less than 1 year), exacerbated by stress, and more distressful to parents than patient. Tics are best treated in two ways. Attempt to alleviate stress and ignore the tic. If tics become chronic, psychotherapy may be indicated. Remember that tics can occur in neurologic disease, too. Tourette's syndrome consists of tics, impulsive behavior, and coprolalia (swearing). Treatment usually includes neuroleptics.

Child Abuse

We've saved the worst for last. Enormous numbers of children are abused physically and sexually every year; the effects of such abuse on the child's personality development are devastating. Physical abuse occurs in all social classes and comes in a myriad of packages including blows, torture, and even murder. Generally, child abuse consists of any behavior within the child's environment that interferes with the child's development.

We can actually be a little more specific. Child abuse results in personality changes, in the child. These children experience a role reversal with their parents. They wind up caring for their own parents. Such abused children sometimes have precocious development. They are expected to behave like adults. For example, they may cook family meals at the age of 6. They may be very aggressive at times, themselves, and when grown up will often abuse their own children. They may also suffer from developmental delays if the abuse has been severe. Such abused children may be unable to empathize with other people. Therefore, they may have difficulty appreciating the effects of violence on others.

Abused children usually are found in families where the parents, themselves, had been abused. These families are often physically isolated. The parents are suspicious of medical care and feel self-righteous in their attitudes about child-rearing. They can be very violent and may need treatment in hospital settings. In spite of abusing their children, they may have extraordinarily high expectations of the children. Occasionally, child abuse is a disorder of neglect; it is usually a disorder of overstimulation of the child.

Recent research has emphasized collusion in child abuse. For example, one parent may dole out the physical abuse while the other "turns his or her back." The colluding parent is aware, consciously or unconsciously, that abuse is occuring, but does nothing to stop it, and may even promote it. The colluding parent is as dangerous to the child as the abusive one.

When you seriously suspect child abuse, you must report it! Report it to the social services agency and then do whatever is necessary to protect the well-being of the child. This can include hospitalization or sending the police to the home to check on the child's safety. Psychiatric treatment should usually consist of psychotherapy for both child and the family. Parental counseling is often necessary but rarely helpful in and of itself.

CHAPTER 11. THE PATIENT WITH SEXUAL PROBLEMS

An open-minded approach to the patient with sexual problems is essential. Such problems are common, arouse great anxiety and concern, and are difficult to discuss. The afflicted patient may not express his or her concerns directly. A veiled question or last-minute comment may be the only clue that the patient has something else to discuss, i.e. a sexual problem. Though discussing sexual dysfunctions may arouse anxiety in the patient as well as the doctor, they should not be overlooked. They have an important differential diagnosis and often cause significant problems in relationships.

Frame your approach with an understanding of normal sexual physiology. Sexual *arousal* (penile erection; vaginal lubrication, engorgement of the labia, vaginal walls, and clitoris) is followed by a *plateau* phase (following intensification of the arousal the physical excitement levels off). Then, orgasm (ejaculation; rhythmic contractions of the perineal and perivaginal muscles) occurs. Women may have multiple orgasms. Men have a refractory period after orgasm during which they are resistant to sexual excitement and cannot ejaculate. This refractory period may last a few minutes to several hours and increases with increasing age. After orgasm, detumescence (loss of both erection and vasocongestion) occurs.

Erection and vaginal lubrication (and the corresponding vasocongestion in both sexes) are parasympathetically mediated. Ejaculation is mediated by the sympathetic nervous system. Therefore, injuries, drugs, or illnesses that interfere with these parts of the nervous system will affect either erection/vasocongestion or ejaculation/orgasm.

After determining the phase(s) in which dysfunction occurs, you can identify the particular sexual dysfunction. Remember: AROUSAL, ORGASM, and KINKY (referring to people who prefer something other than adult-to-adult intercourse). That's A-O.K., a term used by astronauts shot into space.

A: Arousal and Desire Disorders

DSM-IV distinguishes disorders of sexual arousal and sexual desire. Hypoactive sexual desire disorder and sexual aversion disorder are self explanatory.

Disorders of sexual arousal are termed *female sexual arousal disorder and male erectile disorder* (impotence, lifelong and acquired) in DSM-IV. Arousal disorders cause failure to achieve erection or vaginal lubrication.

Lifelong impotence is rare. It refers to the failure to ever achieve an erection. Lifelong impotence is more difficult to treat and the prognosis is worse. It may be associated with a personal history of social withdrawal and isolation. Extreme fear of women is usually a dynamic factor.

Acquired impotence occurs after a period of normal erectile functioning and is the #1 sexual complaint of men.

Let's review the differential diagnosis:

—Endocrine problems cause impotence (pituitary tumors, hyperthyroidism, Addison's disease).

—Medications like antidepressants, anticholinergics, antihypertensives, neuroleptics, and ethanol cause impotence.

—Acute or chronic illness can cause impotence.

—Peripheral neuropathies cause impotence (e.g., associated with diabetes mellitus, alcoholism).

—Trauma to the spinal cord or genital area can lead to impotence.

—Psychological factors may play a role. For example, depression causes a loss of libido. Impotence can occur. Anxiety about sexual performance can be etiologic. Also, marital discord or anger at the sexual partner can cause impotence.

Treat the underlying condition. If a cause can be found, it should be treated. Remember, the same patient may be affected by both psychological and physical factors.

Treat the underlying psychological cause(s). Depression responds to antidepressants and psychotherapy. Marital discord requires marital therapy. Anxiety is treated with psychotherapy and de-emphasis on sexual performance. Some men become spectators to their own sexual performance and can't relax. This causes impotence. Emphasize foreplay, i.e. a focus on the pleasure of the sexual excitement and exploration with the partner, and try to restrict actual intercourse, at first. Then, counsel the patient and his partner to progress gradually to intercourse. Counsel against excessive use of alcohol and refer for alcohol treatment if necessary (see Chapter 8).

Female frigidity has a similar differential diagnosis, but some of the psychological causes are different. Fear of pregnancy or harm may be paramount. A previous sexual assault could have caused a post-traumatic stress disorder. Thinking of or participating in sex could rekindle memories of the assault. Similarly, evidence is growing that significant numbers of females (possibly 1 in 4) may have been sexually abused by male relatives or other males during their childhood. Recollection of the trauma of these experiences may also contribute to this problem. Treatment should be psychotherapy.

O: Orgasm Disorders

The dysfunctions that occur during this phase are premature ejaculation and male orgasmic disorder for men, and female orgasmic disorder for women (DSM-IV).

Premature ejaculation is common and treatable. If the patient ejaculates before he wants to he can be trained to delay ejaculation. Several techniques may be used in sexual treatment to facilitate this. Basically, the sexual activity with the partner is stopped just prior to the point where the man senses ejaculation is imminent. Then, he either receives no stimulation or the glans of the penis is squeezed by the partner. The goal in both approaches is to decrease the arousal. Before detumescence occurs, the sexual activity is resumed until the man again signals the partner to stop. With this start-stop procedure the man and the woman both gain a greater sense of control and the problem diminishes. Anxiety plays a role in premature ejaculation. Therefore, psychotherapy frequently helps.

Male orgasmic disorder (retarded ejaculation) can be due to physical or emotional problems. Antihypertensives, GU surgery, alcohol abuse, and spinal cord damage lead to this condition. Anxiety, sexual deviations (see KINKY), and marital stress also lead to inhibited orgasms. Obviously, treat any underlying condition. Attempt to teach the patient to ejaculate by self-masturbation before encouraging him to participate in intercourse. This helps obviate interpersonal stress that results when the partner feels unattractive and unappealing as a result of the man's failure to reach orgasm.

Female orgasmic disorder should be similarly treated. Since women differ in their responses to genital stimulation, each should be encouraged to explore her responses to a range of forms of stimulation (e.g., clitoral, vaginal, etc.) Psychological causes should be explored and treated (e.g., anxiety, performance anxiety, guilt). Obviously, effective communication between sexual partners is pivotal to successful sex in this and other dysfunctions. Reassurance and encouragement from the primary physician may be helpful. Some problems may be due to a lack of knowledge of sexual functioning. In these cases, books on normal sexual function may be recommended prior to psychotherapy.

The new and widely prescribed antidepressants fluoxetine, sertraline and paroxetine commonly cause orgasmic disorder in both men and women.

K: Kinky Disorders

Kinky is a misnomer, but it's a way of remembering the group of sexual dysfunctions in which intercourse is not the preferred means of sexual gratification. The technical term is paraphilia. Here, we'll discuss exhibitionism, sadomasochism, pedophilia, transvestism, and transsexualism. Patients with these conditions don't seek help themselves unless they feel guilty about their desires. They are referred by courts (pedophiles, exhibitionists) and surgeons (transsexuals seeking sex change surgery). Patients often have more than one paraphilia, e.g. a pedophile may also be an exhibitionist.

Exhibitionists derive sexual gratification (including orgasm) from exposing their genitals. The condition is more common in men who expose themselves to women and scare them. These men achieve unconscious validation that they are "men" by the reactions they obtain. Usually, exhibitionists come to the psychiatrist's attention via court referral. They are difficult to treat, because they deny having the condition and don't want to change. (See Question 47, Chapter 13).

Sadomasochists must hurt or be hurt to obtain sexual gratification. A fusion of sexual and aggressive impulses has occurred. Treatment is prolonged psychotherapy.

Pedophiles obtain sexual gratification by molesting pre-adolescent children. The perpetrator is usually a man. The victim may be a boy or girl. Frightened by secondary sexual characteristics (breasts, pubic hair, etc.), pedophiles seek young children. Treatment is intensive cognitive-behavioral therapy and legal sanctions.

Transvestites are men who are sexually aroused by wearing female clothing. They may also have "normal" heterosexual lives. The etiology is unknown, but traumatic childhood experiences are suspected, e.g., mother forcing her boy to wear female clothing. Treatment is long-term psychotherapy.

Transsexuals want to be members of the opposite sex. The condition is rare in women. A primary transsexual is a man who has always wanted to be a woman. He should have a history of feminine behavior since early childhood. A secondary transsexual desires a sex change after a period of normal gender behavior. Schizophrenics and homosexuals may suffer secondary transsexualism.

The distinction between primary and secondary transsexualism is important. Primary transsexuals don't accept their gender identity. They deny that their genitals can be used for sexual gratification as a male. Their prognosis for psychological change is poor. A sex change operation is indicated if they are adult, failed at psychotherapy to change their attitude, suffer primary transsexualism, and want the surgery. After surgery, their adjustment to life may not improve. Secondary transsexuals should have their underlying condition treated (e.g., chlorpromazine for schizophrenia).

Five to ten percent of the population is homosexual; that is, primarily sexually aroused by members of the same sex. The etiology is debated. Some believe early environmental factors play a role, e.g., a young boy is repeatedly frightened by his father and begins to seek non-aggressive men for gratification of needs to be close to a man. Others consider genetic and biologic influences to be paramount.

Homosexuals can suffer consequences secondary to their sexual preference. They may be scorned or rejected by friends and family. Anxiety and depression may develop and should be treated. Those who have many sexual contacts are at increased risk for certain infectious diseases (e.g., hepatitis, shigella, AIDS). While the psychiatrist won't treat these diseases, he should be aware of the anxiety that they cause.

Rarely, a homosexual will ask for help in changing his/her sexual orientation. Psychotherapy helps some, but behavior modification and counseling are more effective.

CHAPTER 12. PERSONALITY DISORDERS

A personality disorder consists of habitual maladaptive behavior without significant signs or symptoms of other mental illness. A personality disorder should be distinguished from personality traits. Personality traits are behaviors or mannerisms that are habit but aren't pervasive enough to be the full blown personality disorder. Everyone has a personality "style." Only a few have personality disorders.

A personality disorder should slap you in the face. People with these conditions are in frequent trouble with relationships, with the law, or with their work. They are in BAD SHAPE, a mnemonic to help you remember the categories of personality disorders.

Borderline: These patients dread separations. See below for further explanation.

Antisocial: These patients habitually break the law.

Dependent: These are people who rely on others for guidance and emotional support.

Schizoid: These are people who are aloof, withdrawn and difficult to engage.

Schizotypal: These are people who have odd and nearly psychotic mannerisms but aren't fully schizophrenic.

Histrionic: These are people who exaggerate and who respond with strong emotions to relatively minor difficulties.

Avoidant: These are people who show attachment to others but who shy away from social relationships.

Paranoid: In this personality disorder, the patient is suspicious of others but not psychotic.

Passive-Aggressive: Such patients use passivity to express angry feelings. For example, they show up late for an important appointment to express their anger at their doctor.

Empathic disorder: We've fudged here. The real name of this personality disorder is narcissistic personality disorder. However, people with this condition can't empathize; in fact they often become angry if you can't understand them. They are also extremely vain.

Borderline, antisocial, and narcissistic personality disorders will be discussed in greater detail. These are the conditions that most commonly come to physicians' attention.

A *borderline* patient is in BAD SHAPE. He suffers impulsivity (e.g., substance abuse, fighting, gambling), intense rage, unstable affect, recurrent suicide attempts, and fear of being alone. He often has multiple somatic complaints and may be hypochondrical. Most noteworthy, he has unstable interpersonal relationships. These problems are chronic.

Unstable relationships bring these patients to the doctor. Such patients dread being alone; that is, they fear "separation." To avoid separation, they try to coerce others into staying with them. For example, they threaten or attempt suicide when faced with a separation. They quickly attach to and over-value others (e.g., the doctor). They're promiscuous, to get others to be near them.

Borderline patients pose problems for the doctor/patient relationship. Initially these patients over-value the doctor. To control the doctor, they may threaten suicide (e.g., if not granted a request for a prescription). They sometimes attempt to seduce the doctor. When denied their inappropriate wishes, they occasionally sue the doctor. The doctor must behave appropriately towards all patients. If he thinks his patient has a borderline personality disorder, and he is having trouble managing the patient, a referral to a psychiatrist is indicated. If the patient refuses a referral, the doctor has two choices. He can seek psychiatric consultation and attempt to deal with the patient himself. Or, he can decline to treat the patient, if the patient is behaving inappropriately.

Early environmental experiences play a role in the etiology of borderline personality disorder. A child, constantly threatened with abandonment, may grow to fear separations. Some think biological factors play a role, too (e.g., abnormal neurotransmitters).

Treatment is lengthy and complex. In general, the therapist should not yield to coercive efforts by the patient. The therapist must anticipate difficult times for the patient (e.g., the therapist goes on vacation, a separation) and help the patient find new ways of coping with these experiences. The patient will probably require many hospitalizations for suicide ideation or attempt. Drugs are only modestly effective. Occasionally the patient may have psychotic symptoms and neuroleptics may help.

Antisocial personality disorder is characterized by a basic disregard for the rights of others, recurrent law-breaking, and a history of antisocial behavior in childhood (e.g., shoplifting, truancy, fighting at school). Other features of antisocial personality disorder are trouble maintaining employment, trouble being a good parent, multiple divorces, impulsivity, lying, and recklessness (DSM-III-R).

In hospitals, patients with this disorder present with demands for pain medication. Their children may be abused. In society, they break the law repeatedly.

An abnormal superego is characteristic. Pathological parenting causes poor superego development in these patients. For example, a parent who condones rather than limits aggressive behavior in his child, teaches the child that fighting is okay. Genetic factors play a role. Adopted children with an antisocial parent (biological) are at greater risk for this condition. The disorder is probably not more common in men with two Y chromosomes (i.e., XYY), as previously thought. Treatment consists of limiting the antisocial behavior, when possible. This can sometimes be accomplished with a jail term or other social pressure (e.g., taking away custody of children, if they are abused). Patients with antisocial personality disorder have low self-esteem. They also react angrily when confronted. So, the therapist should appear to be particularly interested in these patients (helps self-esteem) and should gently confront lying, stealing, etc.

Narcissistic personality disorder is a relatively new diagnosis, because people with this condition have problems we all can relate to. They like attention and admiration, have a strong sense of self-importance, are sensitive to criticism, and are preoccupied with success and power. However, they also exploit others, have abnormal relationships, and lack empathy. This last symptom is the most important.

The patient with narcissistic personality disorder can't appreciate others' feelings. Furthermore, lack of empathy in the patient's upbringing causes the condition. Growing up in an understanding environment is important for healthy psychological functioning. Unempathic parents cause children to feel lonely, inferior, and misunderstood. To compensate, these children try harder to please others. When they grow up, they become very sensitive to criticism and misunderstanding. They compensate for their sense of inferiority by striving for greatness.

Therefore, they will come to the doctor's office when they have failed to succeed or have been criticized. They will complain of depression, boredom, or empty feelings. They may describe a wish to retaliate with the person who has criticized them. A sense of failure can even lead to suicide attempts.

The treatment is long-term psychotherapy. The therapist will invariably, but certainly not deliberately, misunderstand the patient from time to time. The patient's reactions to this misunderstanding are explored and explained to him. Eventually, such patients come to terms with their vulnerability to criticism.

Remember, a patient with personality disorder is in BAD SHAPE. That means, he is in frequent or constant trouble, and the trouble significantly interferes with his life. It interferes with his social relationship, his work, or his ability to be a law abiding citizen.

CHAPTER 13. TREATMENT MODALITIES

Psychotherapy

Psychotherapy is the form of treatment most people associate with psychiatric care. It's development by Sigmund Freud is described in Chapter 1. It comes in a variety of forms.

Dynamic or *psychoanalytic psychotherapy* attempts to understand intrapsychic conflict. In this form of therapy, symptom relief is obtained as understanding of the conflict proceeds. Dynamic psychotherapy is most useful for patients whose problems are with interpersonal relationships. Symptoms which the patient senses emanate primarily from within himself are also amenable to this treatment. The patient knows that his symptoms or conflicts are unreasonable, but he feels unable to change them by logic, alone. The patient is usually seen once or twice a week and offered the chance to talk about his problems and feelings. The psychiatrist helps out by clarifying conflicts, transferences, and defenses.

Behavioral psychotherapy is based on learning theory. Here, psychological symptoms are considered to be the result of learned or conditioned maladaptive patterns of response. In this form of treatment, a particular behavior or response is identified for the focus of therapeutic intervention. The events which precede this specific behavior (antecedents) are searched for in great detail as are the events which follow the behavior (consequences). The consequences may be understood as either rewarding or punishing in nature. With detailed behavioral analysis of the context of a particular symptom, a treatment strategy may be devised for changing it. Behavioral therapy strategies include systematic desensitization, assertiveness training, and others.

Systematic desensitization is used for the treatment of various phobias and other specific anxiety symptoms. The patient is taught progressive muscle relaxation or another relaxation technique. This procedure involves systematically tensing and relaxing most major muscle groups in the body, sequentially. The focus is on the contrast between the tension and the relaxation experience in each area of the body. With practice, the patient learns to deeply relax using this technique. Basically, this technique of relaxation is then gradually paired with the anxiety-producing stimulus or setting. This may be done with the patient's evoking mental images of progressively more anxiety producing situations. It may also involve actual live experiences of the feared situation. As the situation arrives, the technique of relaxation is used to compete with the anticipated anxiety and therefore replaces it in the patient's experience. Over time, this may lead to significant or complete reduction of anxiety in the feared situation. Desensitization and relaxation are also used in the treatment of some sexual dysfunctions.

Assertiveness training is a technique in which a specific assertive manner is acquired to replace a symptom of fear or anxiety in a particular *social* situation. This may be done in individual therapeutic settings or in group therapeutic settings via role playing. It involves another person playing the fearful person. The patient responds by replacing his usual anxious timidity or withdrawal with an assertive self-confident statement. Alcohol and drugs are frequently used to deal with feared social situations. Consequently, this form of treatment is common in alcohol and drug abuse facilities where patients often have very low self-esteem.

In the past 2 decades new, focused types of psychotherapy have been developed. *Cognitive therapy* was devised to treat depression and other mental disorders by identifying and correcting, in a systematic way, distortions in thinking prevalent in the disorders. Cognitive therapy and *interpersonal psychotherapy of depression* have been shown to be very effective in treating depression in several multicenter studies.

Group and marital psychotherapy is based on behavioral theories, dynamic theories or combinations of the two. Psychotherapy groups may be used to help patients develop social skills and are particularly useful for patients with chronic mental illness. Groups may also provide interpersonal support. This can enhance self-esteem among the members via an awareness that other people suffer from the same symptoms, feelings, and thoughts. When treating children, family or marital therapy can be extremely important in helping alter feelings and behavior which may adversely affect the child.

An important, and at times difficult, decision is the choice of *outpatient* versus *inpatient* psychiatric treatment. The indications for inpatient psychiatric treatment usually include:

1)   suicidal or homicidal behavior related to a psychological problem.

2)   symptoms of significant disorganization of personality functioning such as the inability to feed or clothe oneself adequately.

3)   impulsive self-destructive behavior or inability to control emotional outbursts.

4)   for the purposes of diagnostic evaluation, for example, attempting to determine whether particular disabling psychological symptoms are physiological or psychological in nature.

Inpatient psychiatric treatment includes focused psychotherapy, group and family therapy, occupational therapy, and usually medication.

Antipsychotic Agents

Psychopharmacology has made major advances in the past several decades. The development of chlorpromazine (Thorazine) as an antipsychotic drug in the 1950's began a major change in psychiatric treatment. Since then, the ability to ameliorate many of the symptoms of chronic schizophrenia with chlorpromazine and later drugs has allowed for a drastic reduction of the population in state mental hospitals. These drugs are also called major tranquilizers or neuroleptics. The first family of these drugs was the phenothiazines in which chlorpromazine was followed by trifluoperazine (Stelazine), thioridazine (Mellaril) and fluphenazine (Prolixin). Subsequently, other antipsychotic drugs of somewhat different chemical structures were developed including thiothixene (Navane), haloperidol (Haldol), and others. The primary indication for these drugs is schizophrenia. Other indications may be the manic phase of bipolar disorder; paranoid states; and intoxication with sympathomimetic drugs (such as amphetamines or cocaine), when delusional symptoms resembling acute schizophrenia develop.

In the 1990s a new class of antipsychotic agents has appeared. This group is called 'atypical' because their predominant mechanism of action in the brain does not appear to be the blockade of dopamine (D2) receptors as is the case with the older antipsychotics. While the new drugs act at the D2 site, they also act at multiple other receptors. The first atypical was clozapine (Clozaril). It is as effective as haloperidol, the current antipsychotic benchmark, for the positive symptoms (hallucinations and delusions) of schizophrenia and actually superior to haloperidol for negative symptoms (apathy, withdrawal, flat affect). The next drug in this class, risperidone (Risperdal), was released in recent years and appears to be as effective as haloperidol. Two newer atypicals have been approved by the FDA, olanzapine (Zyprexa) and quetiapine (Seroquel). These agents appear to be equal in efficacy and have a side effect profile that offers some advantages over haloperidol. Clozapine is more effective than haloperidol but a 1% risk of agranulocytosis necessitates an extensive monitoring program by psychiatrists and it is approved only for those patients whose pyschotic illness has been resistant to conventional treatments.

Table 6 lists the equivalent dosages for the older antipsychotic medications and the usual therapeutic dosage range. Table 7 lists the usual starting doses of the atypical antipsychotics and their common dosage ranges.

TABLE 6

Drug	Equivalent (oral) dose	Daily therapeutic dosage range for schizophrenia (approx.)
Chlorpromazine (Thorazine)	100 mg	200–1600 mg
Thioridazine (Mellaril)	100 mg	200– 800 mg*
Trifluoperazine (Stelazine)	5 mg	10– 80 mg
Fluphenazine (Prolixin)	2 mg	5– 40 mg
Thiothixene (Navane)	5 mg	10– 80 mg
Haloperidol (Haldol)	2 mg	5– 40 mg

*May cause pigmentary retinopathy at doses > 800mg/d

TABLE 7

Drug	Usual starting dose	Common dose range
Clozapine	25–50mg bid	150–400mg/d
Risperidone	.5–1mg bid	2–8mg/d
Olanzapine	7.5–10mg hs	10–30mg hs
Quetiapine	25–50mg bid	300–500mg/d

The major side effects of the older antipsychotic drugs include extrapyramidal reactions and anticholinergic effects. The three major extrapyramidal reactions are the dystonias, akathisia, and parkinsonian side effects. Dystonic reactions occur more frequently with high potency neuroleptics (e.g., Haldol), tend to develop early in treatment (first several days), and usually consist of contractions of neck muscles or eye muscles (oculogyric crisis). Akathisia is a subjective symptom of extreme inner restlessness and inability to sit still. It tends to develop several days or weeks after instituting therapy. Pseudoparkinsonism consists of cogwheel rigidity, pill rolling tremor of the hands, mask-like facial expression, and shuffling gait, which occur one to several weeks after starting treatment and are more common with high potency neuroleptics. Anticholinergic side effects include dry mouth, blurred vision, urinary retention, constipation, dry skin and mucous membranes, delirium, and acute glaucoma. Rarely, the central anticholinergic syndrome may occur in which the patient becomes delirious and experiences severe (and life-threatening) autonomic instability. It may seem paradoxical, but anticholinergic drugs are used to treat the extra-pyramidal symptoms. Physostigmine can be used to counteract anticholinergic poisoning.

Tardive dyskinesia is an unusual extrapyramidal side effect of antipsychotic drugs. It usually consists of spontaneous movements of the face including rolling the tongue, smacking the lips, and chewing or blowing motions. Less commonly, movements of the trunk or limbs resembling chorea or tics occur. The disorder may begin after only a few months on these medications but more often occurs after several years at relatively high doses. It may be an irreversible side effect.

Other side effects of the neuroleptics include jaundice, leukopenia, pigmentary retinopathy (with thioridazine), and pigment deposits in the skin and the lens of the eye.

The atypical antipsychotics, particularly olanzapine and/or quetiapine, may soon become the drugs of choice for most psychotic disorders. They appear to cause fewer extrapyramidal side effects than the older drugs and may pose less of a risk for tardive dyskinesia. Risperidone appears to be more activating and is likely to be weight neutral. Olanzapine and quetiapine are more sedating and olanzapine can cause significant weight gain. Quetiapine has been reported to be associated with the development of cataracts in some laboratory animals, and a conservative recommendation is for slit lamp exams before and during the treatment with this agent. An additional concern with the newer agents is their high cost. However, this may be balanced by better patient compliance with lower overall morbidity leading to fewer hospital days, improved personal relationships, and a greater chance of maintaining employment.

For the emergency treatment of most acute psychotic conditions haloperidol remains the drug of choice.

Antidepressants

There are three main classes of antidepressant drugs, the tricyclics and the MAO (monoamine oxidase) inhibitors and the selective serotonin reuptake inhibitors (SSRIs). *Imipramine (Tofranil),* the first tricyclic antidepressant, was developed in the late 1950's. Since that time, *amitriptyline (Elavil), doxepin (Sinequan), desipramine (Norpramin)* and others have been developed. A proposed mechanism for the effectiveness of these drugs is based on their effect on the release, uptake, or metabolism of norepinephrine or serotonin in the central nervous system. Although many new drugs of this class have been developed, there has yet to be conclusive proof that any of the newer drugs is significantly more effective than imipramine in treating randomly selected patients with severe depression.

The SSRIs have become the first line agents for both major depression and dysthymia. They are also indicated for panic disorder and obsessive compulsive disorder. Fluoxetine (Prozac) was introduced in 1988 and is now the most widely prescribed antidepressant in the country. The favorable side effect profile of these drugs and their relative safety and simplicity have led to their rapid rise. The SSRIs are neither anticholinergic nor antihistaminic. Therefore, dry mouth, constipation, blurred vision, urinary retention, sedation, and weight gain are uncommon. All of the SSRIs may cause nausea, tension headaches, increased anxiety, insomnia (though paradoxically they may cause daytime drowsiness), and sexual dysfunction (here we go again). Decreased libido, anorgasmia in women, and retarded ejaculation in men may occur in 20–40% of patients. Yohimbine, cyproheptadine, or bethanocol may be helpful for this side effect. The SSRIs are not cardiotoxic and are rarely, if ever, lethal in overdose when no other drugs are involved. Overall, however, only 10–15% of patients discontinue these agents due to side effects. Dosing is once daily for fluoxetine, sertraline (Zoloft), and paroxetine (Paxil) and once or twice daily for fluvoxamine (Luvox). Table 8 lists the usual dose ranges and side effect comparisons. The starting dose is usually 1/2 the lowest dose, listed in Table 8, for one week. Then it is raised to the lowest usual dose, e.g. 20mg of fluoxetine, for 4–5 weeks. The patient's response is then reevaluated and the dose is adjusted as needed.

The initial dosage of tricyclic antidepressant should be 25-50 mg/d. It should be increased by 25mg every 3-4 days until the therapeutic dosage is reached. Patients usually begin to respond within two weeks of reaching the therapeutic dose; how-

TABLE 8

Drug	Usual effective therapeutic dosage	Sedation	Antianxiety effects	Anticholinergic effects
Imipramine	150–200mg/d	+ +	+	+ +
Amitriptyline	150–200mg/d	+ + + +	+ +	+ + + +
Doxepin	150–200mg/d	+ + +	+ +	+ + +
Desipramine	150–200mg/d	+	0	+
Fluoxetine (Prozac)	20–60mg/d	+	+	0
Paroxetine (Paxil)	20–50mg/d	+	+	±
Sertraline (Zoloft)	50–200mg/d	+	+	0
Fluvoxamine (Luvox)	50–300mg/d	+	+	0

ever, response occasionally takes up to six weeks. In older people, antidepressants should be used cautiously, as they (like many drugs) may be metabolized more slowly, thus increasing the risk of toxicity. The danger of falling due to orthostatic hypotension calls for lower initial dosages and a slower increase in dose in this age group. Other side effects of the tricyclics may include anticholinergic and antihistamine symptoms. Cardiac arrhythmias (most commonly prolonged PR interval, but also more serious abnormalities) are possible, and this is the primary reason that the tricyclics may be lethal in overdose. These drugs are metabolized in the liver and jaundice has occurred rarely.

The MAO inhibitors are also effective antidepressants. However, in addition to affecting norepinephrine and serotonin in the central nervous system, they also affect the metabolism of tyramine. A build-up of tyramine could lead to a hypertensive crisis if excess tyramine were ingested (in cheese, beer, beans, yeast). Sympathomimetic drugs (tricyclics, ephedrine, L-dopa, decongestants) may potentiate the MAO inhibitors' hypertensive effects. For this reason, psychiatrists have been cautious about using these drugs. Recent research has suggested that this class of drugs is effective in treating severe depressions and panic disorders. Major MAO inhibitor drugs include phenelzine (Nardil), isocarboxazide (Marplan), and tranylcypromine (Parnate).

Other useful antidepressants, not in the major classes are trazodone (Desyrel), nefazodone (Serzone), maprotilene (Ludiomil), buproprion (Wellbutrin), venlafaxine (Effexor) and mirtazapine (Remeron). Trazodone affects the serotonergic receptors, is quite sedating, but minimally anticholinergic, and less dangerous in overdose than the tricyclics. Maprotilene and buproprion are not sedating and induce minimal weight gain but are associated with a greater risk of seizures than other agents. Bupropion and venlafaxine have recently been reformulated in sustained release preparations, Wellbutrin SR and Effexor XR, respectively. The sustained release bupropion, dosed at 150mg bid, has also been shown in controlled trials to be effective in smoking cessation in about 60% of patients and has been marketed under a new trade name, Zyban. Interestingly some managed care companies, with their questionable value systems, are refusing to pay for this drug for smoking cessation. In response to this, some clinicians are prescribing the antidepressant form, Wellbutrin SR, which is more often covered by insurance.

Clomipramine (Anafranil) was the first medication approved for the treatment of obsessive compulsive disorder (OCD). It is a first generation tricyclic with a side effect profile similar to amitriptyline. All of the SSRIs have now received indications by the FDA for OCD and are the first choice for this condition due to their favorable side effect profiles. Effective treatment for OCD usually requires dosages in the higher end of the accepted range.

The treatment of panic disorder may include cognitive-behavioral therapy and one of several antidepressants. Imipramine was first used for panic in the 1960s and it is still used for this indication. The MAO inhibitors are often very effective but their use is limited due to the potential adverse reactions cited above. The SSRIs have become a first line treatment for panic disorder and, though higher doses are sometimes required, occasionally patients respond to one-half of the usual dose.

Mood Stabilizers

Lithium carbonate is a salt that was found to be useful in treating manic-depressive illness. Specifically, lithium is effective in the treatment of the manic phase of illness and is secondarily useful in the prevention of manic episodes. To a lesser degree it may prevent depressive episodes. The usual effective dosage range of lithium carbonate is 600-2400mg daily. The actual monitoring of the effective dose is done by checking blood levels, which usually should range from 0.7 to 1.2 meq/L. The exact mechanism by which lithium works is unknown. In patients who are acutely manic the therapeutic effect of lithium is not observed for at least one week, and during that time the use of antipsychotic drugs for behavioral control may be necessary, as well as lithium levels up to 1.5 meq/L.

The side effects of lithium include gastrointestinal symptoms such as nausea, vomiting, diarrhea and indigestion. These can occur at therapeutic blood levels. Dividing doses helps alleviate these symptoms. Toxic effects of lithium include tremors, ataxia, nystagmus, stupor and coma. These symptoms usually occur at blood levels over 1.5 meq/L but in some patients may occur at blood levels significantly less than this. Lithium may also cause cardiac arrhythmias. Increased thirst and polyuria are extremely common side effects of lithium treatment. Long-term use of lithium has been associated with decreased urine concentrating ability and hypothyroidism. When considering patients for long-term lithium use, periodic evaluations of kidney and thyroid function should be performed.

The anticonvulsants, carbamazepine (Tegretol), valproic acid (Depakene), and divalproex sodium (Depakote), have been used in recent years as alternatives to lithium. A recent major multicenter study has demonstrated the efficacy of divalproex sodium in the treatment of the manic phase of bipolar disorder. Studies also show promise for the drug in the treatment of bipolar depression and in the maintenance phase of the disorder. Though carbamazepine has long been used in this population the evidence for its efficacy is equivocal. Several other newer anticonvulsants have been reported to be helpful in bipolar patients including gabapentin (Neurontin) and lamotrigine (Lamictal). Studies are underway with these agents at present.

Sedative-Hypnotics; Antianxiety Agents

The sedative-hypnotics as a group are often called antianxiety drugs or minor tranquilizers. The barbiturates were the first, followed by meprobamate (Equanil), hydroxyzine (Atarax), and chlordiazeproxide (Librium). The benzodiazepines, of which chlordiazepoxide (Librium) was the first, are by far the most widely used drugs of this class at the present time. The utility of these drugs lies primarily in the treatment of short-term circumscribed anxiety and insomnia using the lowest effective dose for the shortest period of time possible. Practically speaking, this means the use of 30 mg per day of diazepam (Valium) or less for no more than 2-3 weeks. Of course, these drugs are also useful in the treatment of alcohol withdrawal. A new relative of the benzodiazepines, alprazolam (Xanax), has been shown to be useful in patients with panic disorders. However patients rapidly develop a tolerance to alprazolam. There is a fine line between the clear potential for abuse of drugs in this class and their effectiveness for certain symptoms. Judicious use of these drugs in the manner prescribed is not likely to lead to dependence.

Buspirone (Buspar) was introduced for the treatment of generalized anxiety some years ago. It is unrelated to the benzodiazepines and is not addictive. Many patients who have previously taken a benzodiazepine complain that it is ineffective. In fact, it can be quite useful in certain patients but its onset of action is similar to the antidepressants, 2-6 weeks, so the patient must be reassured. The usual starting dose is 7.5mg bid; the dose is then titrated upward to 15-30mg bid. Common side effects are dizziness and nausea which usually disappear within a few weeks.

Zolpidem (Ambien) is a new sedative agent which is very similar to the benzodiazepines. It has a rapid onset of action and usually little residual morning drowsiness. Tolerance develops to the drug so brief or very intermittent use is indicated. It shares side effects with the benzodiazepines including, rarely, antero-grade amnesia.

Adjunctive Medications for Alcohol Treatment

Disulfiram (Antabuse) is a drug that can be an effective adjunct in the treatment of alcoholism. If the patient drinks alcohol after having taken this drug, he will have an alcohol-Antabuse reaction. The reaction consists of skin flushing, ele-vated pulse rate, increased respiration, hypotension, chest pain, nausea, copious vomiting, diaphoresis and blurred vision. Severe reactions may lead to respiratory depression, cardiovascular collapse, cardiac arrhythmias, congestive heart failure, seizures and death. The drug is therefore useful only in those patients who sin-cerely wish to stop drinking and may be likely to drink on impulse. The usual dose range is 250mg-500mg daily. The drug is only an adjunct to a comprehensive al-cohol treatment approach as outlined in Chapter 8.

Naltrexone (Revia; Trexan), an opiate antagonist/agonist, was originally de-veloped for the treatment of opiate dependence. It was recently approved by the FDA to aid in the treatment of alcohol dependence. Studies have shown that nal-trexone reduces the craving for alcohol in some patients. It may also reduce the euphoric effects of alcohol, leading to decreased consumption of alcohol when a patient does drink. The usual dose is 25-50mg HS. As with disulfiram, naltrex-one is only an adjunctive agent and a potential part of the approach outlined in Chapter 8.

Electroconvulsive Therapy

Electroconvulsive therapy (ECT) is the most maligned treatment modality in psychiatry. It consists of strategically placing electrodes on the scalp (either in the temporal region bilaterally or one electrode at the vertex of the scalp and the other at the temporal region on the non-dominant side). Then, a precisely mea-sured electrical impulse is passed through the brain. This causes a generalized convulsive seizure. Pre-treatment with a short-acting barbiturate, such as sodium thiopental, and a short-acting muscle relaxant, such as succinylcholine, is neces-sary. This allows the patient to experience only a very short-term general anes-thesia and a significant diminution of the tonic-clonic movements in the generalized seizure. Therapeutic response is correlated with total seizure time. Following the treatment, the patient is post-ictal. He or she is confused, disori-ented to time, and sometimes place. The patient may have a headache and some muscular pains. These symptoms last only a few hours. The most troublesome side effect is short-term memory loss, which lasts several hours to several days. Rarely, patients will complain of long-term memory problems. The use of unilat-eral ECT with the electrical current passing through the non-dominant hemisphere reduces the degree of memory loss. The efficacy of ECT in severe depression is considerable, with eighty percent or more of patients with severe depressions having a markedly positive response. A controversy surrounds the aesthetics of this treatment and its potential for abuse. Consequently, ECT is mainly used in patients who have not responded to adequate trials of several antidepressants, patients who have had a positive response to ECT in the past, or patients who are in life-threatening situations. For example, patients who are imminently suicidal (and depressed) or severely catatonic (and not eating or drinking) may not be able to wait for medications to take effect.

CHAPTER 14. CLINICAL REVIEW

It's time to test your knowledge of psychiatry. We hope that the previous chapters have made this specialty more comprehensible! Here we go.

(1) Question: A 25-year-old woman complains of lower back pain. She also appears depressed. How should you evaluate her?

      A) Ask her about other symptoms of depression.
      B) Evaluate her back pain; ignore the depression.
      C) Evaluate her depression; ignore the back pain.
      D) Refer her to a psychiatrist.

Answer: A. Other symptoms of depression include the vegetative signs and suicidal ideation. Her back pain should be seriously evaluated. It could be a depressive equivalent or an organic problem. A referral to a psychiatrist might be appropriate. However, if she is suicidal, it's not safe to let her out of your office until a disposition is arranged. Remember, many people who suicide have seen their primary care physician in the preceding several weeks.

(2) Question: The patient is chronically depressed, but not suicidal. Should you refer her to a psychiatrist?

Answer: Not necessarily. Many patients prefer treatment from their primary care physician. They are reluctant to accept a psychiatric referral or diagnosis.

(3) Question: Should you start this woman on antidepressant medication?

Answer: Probably, if supportive care is ineffective. Make sure she is not allergic to antidepressants. Pregnancy precludes the use of antidepressants. Then begin with 25mg of sertraline for 4-6 days, and then increase to 50mg. If there is no response after 4 weeks, increase to 100mg. Alternatively, begin with a daily dose of 50mg of imipramine. Increase the daily dose by 25mg, every other day. An average daily therapeutic dose of 150mg to 250mg is usually required. The lethal dose of antidepressants is low. Therefore, prescribe it cautiously. Depressed outpatients should be seen several times a week to monitor their symptoms.

(4) Question: Ten days later, the patient is still depressed. What should your next action be?

      A) Change medication.
      B) Stop medication.
      C) Continue medication.
      D) Recommend ECT.

Answer: C.   Antidepressants relieve symptoms of depression after 2-4 weeks. Continue medicating the patient. If treatment fails, change to another antidepressant.

(5) Question: The patient is better. How long should you continue her antidepressants?

Answer: Continue the medication for 6-8 months. Taper antidepressants, because some patients develop withdrawal symptoms (nausea, insomnia, irritability). Follow the patient every other week for 2-3 more months.

(6) Question: A 35-year-old severely depressed woman has been hospitalized and on antidepressant medication for 10 days. She suddenly becomes more pleasant, more organized, pays her 2-month-old doctor's bill, and arranges her affairs at home through a relative who is living there. She comes to you and asks for a pass to leave the hospital. Should you let her go?

Answer: Probably not. When depressed patients appear brighter, happier, more organized, and in charge of their affairs, it can be a sign that they secretly decided to commit suicide. You would want to do a very careful suicide evaluation and observe the patient before making any decision to let her leave the hospital. Of course, your treatment may be working, but antidepressants usually take two to four weeks to take effect. Suicide is more common early in treatment, when patients have increased energy from the medication but still feel hopeless.

(7) Question: A 22-year-old woman has had symptoms of anxiety and depression intermittently for the last five years. After one year of psychotherapy, she develops a transient paralysis of her left arm the morning after taking a sleeping pill. What is your differential diagnosis?

Answer: She could have acute intermittent porphyria, which causes psychological symptoms, neuropathies, and abdominal pain. Porphyria often follows ingestion of barbiturate. She could have a conversion disorder, and this would be corroborated by the psychological findings of previous history of conversion symptoms, identifying with a relative who had a similar symptom, and an immediate (recent) psychological stressor. She also could have both a psychiatric condition and a neurologic condition.

(8) Question: A 20-year-old man is angry at his college professor for giving him a weekend assignment. Shortly after growing angry, he faints. What's wrong with him?

Answer: He could have suffered a conversion symptom. He also could have narcolepsy. Remember, in this disorder, cataplexy (loss of motor tone in response to a strong emotion), may be accompanied by hypnogogic hallucinations, sleep paralysis, and daytime drowsiness.

(9) Question: A 39-year-old woman complains of fatigue and trouble falling asleep. What should you do to evaluate her?

Answer: Do a history, physical exam, and mental status exam. Remember JOIMAT and DEEP.

(10) Question: The mental status exam on this patient shows auditory hallucinations, disorientation, and memory impairment. What is the most likely diagnosis?

   A) Schizophrenia.
   B) Delirium or Dementia.
   C) Depression.
   D) Narcolepsy.

Answer: The answer is B. Delirium is characterized by disorientation, and memory impairment is a key feature of dementia. Hallucinations and delusions can also occur in a delirium.

(11) Question: A work-up for physiologic causes of the patient's symptoms is negative. Could she have a psychiatric illness?

Answer: Yes. Sometimes depression causes disorientation and memory impairment. This is termed *pseudodementia.*

(12) Question: How many psychiatrists does it take to change a light bulb?

Answer: It only takes one, but the light bulb has to want to change. On the surface, this seems a simple joke. In fact, it really is hard to get patients to change their behavior or alter their symptoms if they aren't willing to participate in the treatment themselves.

(13) Question: A 22-year-old schizophrenic patient is admitted with a worsening of his psychotic symptoms and tardive dyskinesia. What is your differential diagnosis?

Answer: He probably has schizophrenia and a tardive dyskinesia. Tardive dyskinesias are late sequelae of neuroleptic treatment. They are motor movements (usually about the mouth and face) that are often irreversible. He also could have Huntington's chorea. Remember, in this illness, schizophrenia-like symptoms can precede the development of the choreiform movements. Wilson's disease causes mental status changes and extrapyramidal signs and symptoms. Don't assume that a patient who appears schizophrenic has schizophrenia. The differential diagnosis is important.

(14) Question: A 65-year-old business man develops auditory hallucinations, paranoia, and anxiety. What is the most likely diagnosis?

   A) Schizophrenia.
   B) Bipolar Disorder.

C) Delirium/Dementia.

D) Sleep apnea.

Answer: C. Schizophrenia begins before age 45. Manic-depressive illness can start late in life. However, the primary problem is an altered mood. Delirium involves disorientation, memory impairment denotes dementia, and psychotic symptoms (hallucinations, paranoia) may accompany either.

(15) Question: In which condition(s) is the risk for suicide increased?

A) Depression.

B) Alcoholism.

C) Anorexia Nervosa.

D) Schizophrenia.

Answer: The suicide risk is increased in all these conditions. Remember SUICIDAL.

(16) Question: A 14-year-old girl lost 30 pounds and now weighs 80 pounds. Medical history, physical exam, and laboratory tests, including electrolytes, are normal. How best do you proceed?

A) Diagnose anorexia nervosa and refer her to a psychiatrist.

B) Tell her she needs to gain weight.

C) No intervention is necessary.

D) Diagnose anorexia nervosa and treat her yourself.

Answer: B. Remember LOW FORM. This patient has *L*oss *o*f *W*eight. Look for *F*ear of *O*besity, *R*efusal to eat, and *M*iscellaneous symptoms. Tell her she needs to gain weight and see if she complies. If she *Refuses* to try to gain weight, its diagnostic of anorexia nervosa.

(17) Question: The patient refuses to eat. What should you do next?

A) Refer her to a psychiatrist.

B) Treat her yourself.

C) Have her sign an AMA (against medical advice) form.

D) Threaten her with hospitalization.

Answer: A. Psychiatrists should help treat these patients.

(18) Question: What is the differential diagnosis of enuresis?

Answer: CAP'IM! CNS, anatomical, psychological, infectious, and metabolic problems can cause enuresis.

(19) Question: How do you evaluate a 7-year-old enuretic boy?

Answer: Look for psychological causes (anger, ambition). Check a urinalysis (to rule out juvenile onset diabetes mellitus, urinary tract infection, and kidney disease). Do not perform an invasive procedure (e.g., cystoscopy) until other causes are excluded.

(20) Question: Should a 7-year-old fire-setter be referred to a child psychiatrist?

Answer: Yes! Fire-setting is serious antisocial behavior. Psychiatric treatment is necessary.

(21) Question: Is somnambulism (sleep walking) safe?

Answer: No. Make sure the somnambulist's room has locked windows and no obstacles.

(22) Question: What condition(s) can be treated with imipramine?
  A) Enuresis.
  B) Depression.
  C) Seizures.
  D) Encopresis (soiling).

Answer: A, B, and C.   Antidepressants have anticholinergic properties. Bladder capacity increases; enuresis usually stops. Antidepressants increase CNS catecholamines. Catecholamine depletion causes depression. Antidepressants may function as neurotransmitters. Imipramine has a limited role in the treatment of seizure disorders. It may lower the seizure threshold, too.

(23) Question: What condition(s) can be treated with amphetamines?
  A) Attention Deficit Disorder with hyperactivity.
  B) Depression.
  C) Obesity.
  D) Narcolepsy.

Answer: A, B, and D.   Amphetamines transiently elevate mood. They may work in treatment resistant depression, particularly in the elderly. Anorexia is a side effect of amphetamines. However, their use in obesity is dangerous.

(24) Question: A 22-year-old man develops a delusion. He believes that Jay Leno wants him to be a guest host on the Tonight Show. How would you characterize this delusion?
  A) Paranoid.
  B) Grandiose.
  C) Realistic.
  D) Somatic.

Answer: B.

(25) Question: What is the most likely diagnosis for this man?

Answer: Schizophrenia. Other symptoms of schizophrenia are hallucinations, catatonia, and loose associations!

(26) Question: A 20-year-old man believes that the FBI wants to hurt him. What kind of delusion is this?

Answer: Paranoid.

(27) Question: The same 20-year-old man denies hallucinations. What is the most likely diagnosis in his case?

Answer: Delusional disorder. Paranoid delusions without hallucinations, catatonia, or loose associations indicates delusional disorder! Otherwise, the diagnosis is schizophrenia.

(28) Question: Which of the following statements is most true about Sigmund Freud?

A) He was a famous baseball player for the New York Mets.
B) He conducts a famous symphony.
C) He was a neurologist.
D) He writes the gourmet section for a famous newspaper.

Answer: C. He was a neurologist. Is that surprising? Modern psychiatry and psychoanalysis actually were an outgrowth of neurology. In the latter part of this century, psychiatry has become a separate specialty, but it appears to be moving closer to neurology and the "medical" sciences.

(29) Question: A 40-year-old chronic schizophrenic man has had a fixed delusion that the telephone wires are talking to him for 15 years. He has also heard voices commenting on his behavior for 10 years. In the last month, he has developed visual hallucinations of spiders crawling down his wall. He now believes the television is talking to him. Why have his symptoms changed?

Answer: Psychotic symptoms tend to remain stable over time. If a schizophrenic patient has a change of symptoms, suspect the possibility that another condition is causing the new psychotic symptoms. He could have a delirium or dementia (he has visual hallucinations, now), a brain tumor, or a worsening of the schizophrenic condition.

(30) Question: A 35-year-old woman with chronic schizophrenia was readmitted to the state hospital with an exacerbation of her chronic paranoid symptoms. She briefly mentioned complaints of occasionally seeing snakes and difficulty concentrating. Her doctor increased her antipsychotic meds, but her symptoms persisted. What's missing here?

Answer: JOIMAT—Review of patient's records revealed that *I*ntellectual function was WNL one year previously and *T*hought content had contained no hallucinations of snakes. *O*n testing, serial 7's and digit span were done poorly; *M*emory was impaired (2/4 objects / 5 min). The patient was referred to a neurologist, who suggested a CT scan. The scan revealed a large temporal lobe tumor. Key points: always do a mental status examination! Change in symptom patterns and new deficits on mental status examinations suggest organic impairment.

(31) Question: A 25-year-old woman develops a delusion that she runs the world. Mental status exam reveals no hallucinations, loose associations, or cognitive impairment. What is her most likely diagnosis?

Answer: Bipolar Disorder (manic phase). *Grandiose* delusions accompany manic-depressive illness. A mood disturbance (euphoria or depression) is usually prominent. However, grandiosity can precede the mood change.

(32) Question: The next day, her mood is very elevated. How should you treat her?
    A) Lithium, as an outpatient.
    B) Lithium, as an inpatient.
    C) Antidepressants.
    D) ECT.

Answer: B. Bipolar patients can become psychotic and agitated quickly. It is best to admit these patients if possible. Lithium is the treatment for this illness. It takes 7-10 days to take action. Neuroleptics (e.g., haloperidol, chlorpromazine) are also effective. They work in 2-3 days but have more serious side effects (e.g., tardive dyskinesia). They are often used until the Lithium takes effect.

(33) Question: A 25-year-old man insists he has cancer of the bowel. A medical work-up does not substantiate his concern. The rest of his mental status exam is WNL. What is his most likely diagnosis?
    A) Delirium/Dementia
    B) Conversion Disorder.
    C) Paranoia.
    D) Depression.

Answer: D. Depression can cause *somatic* delusions. Conversion disorders cause loss or alteration of neurologic functioning. Paranoia causes paranoid delusions. Dementia involves memory impairment, and disorientation accompanies delirium.

(34) Question: A middle-aged man was rushed to a hospital where he had a cardiac arrest. The EKG returned to normal several hours after resuscitation. Coronary angiography and treadmill EKG were normal. The patient gave a history of spontaneous episodes of hyperventilation, tachycardia with fear, and sweating, all occurring several times per week. Was this a yogi who had developed control of his autonomic nervous system to the point that he could stop his heart?

Answer: No. This is a patient with panic disorder (anxiety attacks). Arrhythmias can cause panic attacks. Don't tell these patients "it's all in your head." Many can benefit from SSRIs, tricyclics,

MAO inhibitors, or alprazolam and should be referred to a psychiatrist and internist for further evaluation.

(35) Question: The patient is a well-dressed 40-year-old woman whom you have been treating for manic-depressive illness with lithium. When she arrives for her monthly medication follow-up at 9:00 AM, you wonder if you smell alcohol on her breath. You fear offending the patient with a question regarding alcohol use. What should you do?

Answer: Ask directly, with a concerned rather than confrontive tone, "have you had a drink this morning?" She may be relieved to share her concern over her problem and ask for help. Remember, alcoholism is common in patients with affective disorders.

(36) Question: A 46-year-old reserved and conservative business man suffers a personality change over the course of 6 months. He becomes garrulous, spends a lot of money, and has several sexual affairs. What is your differential diagnosis?

Answer: The first illness to consider is bipolar disorder. It can present at this age and manifests with grandiosity and elevated mood. He could be abusing drugs. Cocaine causes grandiosity, hypersexuality, and similar symptoms. Next, brain tumors can cause personality changes. Last, he could be having a mid-life crisis.

(37) Question: Which mental illness has the best prognosis?
A) Schizophrenia.
B) Bipolar Disorder.
C) Paranoia.

Answer: B. Between episodes, 70% of Bipolar patients function well (e.g., have families and job). Usually, schizophrenia and paranoia are chronic diseases.

(38) Question: How should you treat a 40-year-old Valium addict?
A) Hospitalize and immediately stop all medications.
B) Hospitalize and wean him from his Valium.
C) Gradually reduce his Valium. No need to hospitalize.
D) Start him on methadone.

Answer: B. Abrupt sedative withdrawal can cause tachycardia, hypertension, delirium, and seizures. The best treatment is hospitalization to taper the dose of the sedative.

(39) Question: What causes Kayser-Fleischer rings?
Answer: Wilson's disease. These are copper deposits in the cornea.

(40) Question: Why should a psychiatrist know this?
Answer: Wilson's disease also causes psychiatric symptoms.

(41) Question: A 30-year-old schizophrenic is started on Haldol. He develops torticollis (an extrapyramidal side-effect of neuroleptics). Cogentin (anticholinergic) is used to treat this symptom. Two days later, he develops a fever, tachycardia, blurred vision, and visual hallucinations. How should you treat him?

    A) Stop the Haldol and Cogentin.
    B) Give him more Cogentin.
    C) Give him more Haldol.
    D) Give him Valium.

Answer: A. He has anticholinergic symptoms. These include dry mouth, blurred vision, elevated temperature, and delirium. The medications that have anticholinergic properties should be stopped. It is also important to consider the neuroleptic malignant syndrome, which is treated with supportive care and by withholding neuroleptics, in conjunction with a neurologist.

(42) Question: A 30-year-old schizophrenic man is medicated with Haldol, 30mg per day. On the 10th day of treatment, he becomes catatonic. What should you do?

    A) Increase his Haldol.
    B) Administer ECT.
    C) Decrease his Haldol.
    D) Make no changes in his treatment.

Answer: C. Neuroleptics occasionally cause catatonia. When a patient is medicated with a neuroleptic and develops catatonia, the medication should be stopped. This is a diagnostic maneuver. If the catatonia stops, it probably is due to the neuroleptic.

(43) Question: How do antipsychotic medications work?

    A) They are dopamine agonists.
    B) They are dopamine antagonists.
    C) They block the re-uptake of catacholamines.
    D) They have anticholinergic properties.

Answer: B. Antipsychotic medications are dopamine antagonists. Although they have anticholinergic properties, this does not affect psychoses.

(44) Question: A 25-year-old man is admitted with a 3-week history of auditory hallucinations, delusions, and confusion. What diagnoses are consistent with this clinical presentation?

    A) Amphetamine psychosis.
    B) Schizophreniform psychosis.
    C) Schizophrenia.
    D) Generalized anxiety.

Answer: A and B. Remember, amphetamines can cause psychosis. Schizophrenia psychosis is diagnosed when disorganized or psychotic symptoms have been present less than 6 months. It has a better prognosis than schizophrenia.

(45) Question: What should you do first for this man?

    A) Medicate with an antipsychotic.

    B) Medicate with a sedative (e.g., Valium).

    C) History and physical exam.

    D) Seclude.

Answer: C. Do a history and physical. Look for signs of amphetamine ingestion (dilated pupils, elevated vital signs). Seclude only if the patient is an imminent danger to himself or others on the ward.

(46) Question: The history and physical are normal. When would you prescribe an antipsychotic?

Answer: When possible, it's better to wait for a few days. See if the patient calms down on the ward. His hallucinations and delusions may resolve spontaneously. Medicate him sooner if his psychotic symptoms are causing him to be combative, suicidal, or disruptive. Remember, he could have taken other drugs that can cause a psychosis. If he took an anticholinergic drug, don't prescribe antipsychotics. This class of drugs has anticholinergic properties.

(47) Question: A 25-year-old man is caught exposing his genitals to women in a grocery store. Which answer best explains the etiology of this behavior?

    A) He comes from a low socioeconomic background.

    B) The frightened responses he gets from exposing himself may prove to him that he hasn't been castrated.

    C) He has passive-dependent problems. He is making perverted sexual advances, hoping a woman will respond sympathetically and take care of him.

    D) He has a defect in neurotransmitter synthesis.

Answer: B. *Exhibitionists* achieve sexual gratification by exposing themselves to women. They may have unconscious castration anxiety. When women are frightened, exhibitionists feel better, because it proves to them that they have genitals. Exhibitionists also usually have angry feelings for women.

(48) Question: What does it mean when people say, "a stitch in time saves nine?"

    A) A stitch now will save you a lot of sewing later.

    B) A stitch is a twitch that will stretch the material.

    C) don't procrastinate. A little work now can save a lot of work later.

    D) My stitches got pulled out by the doctor. He put 10 in, and I won at the horse track.

Answer: C. A. is an example of a concrete answer, seen in people who have intellectual trouble with abstractions, or who have a dementia. B. shows clanging associations, seen in mania. D. shows loose and idiosyncratic associations.

(49) Question: A 30-year-old schizophrenic man complains that he does not ejaculate with orgasm. Is this a delusion?

Answer: No. Antipsychotic medications occasionally cause retrograde ejaculation. Thioridazine (Mellaril) is notorious for this side effect. Explain this possible side effect to patients before prescribing the medicine.

(50) Question: A 20-year-old man wants a sex change operation. Which psychiatric condition is occasionally an indication for this surgery?

A) Schizophrenia.
B) Primary transexualism.
C) Secondary transexualism.
D) Homosexuality with feminine characteristics.

Answer: B. A primary transexual has always felt himself to be a woman. He should have a history of feminine behavior since early childhood. His mental status exam should be normal.

PSYCHIATRIC EVALUATION

A-O.K. (disorders of sexual function): Arousal; Orgasm; Kinky.

BAD SHAPE (types of personality disorders): Borderline; Antisocial; Dependent; Schizotypal, Schizoid; Histrionic, Avoidant; Paranoid, Passive aggressive; Empathetic failure (narcissistic).

CAP'IM (causes of enuresis): Central nervous system problems; Anatomical derangements; Psychological; Infections; Metabolic conditions.

DEEP (causes of sleep disturbance): Drugs; Environment; Emotional; Physical.

JOIMAT (mental status exam): Judgement; Orientation; Intellectual functioning; Memory; Affect, Appearance; Thought content.

LOW FORM (findings in anorexia nervosa): Loss Of Weight; Fear of Obesity; Refusal to eat; Miscellaneous.

MED CL (medical problems that parade as psychiatric syndromes): Metals; Endocrine; Drugs; Cancer; Lots of others.

SUICIDAL (suicide risk factors): Sex; Unsuccessful previous attempts; Identification with family history; Chronic Illness; Depression; Age, Alcohol; Lethality of suicidal method; recent Losses.

VACUUM (correlates of childhood anti-social behavior): Violence in family; Alcoholism in family; Child abuse; Unempathetic parenting; Underpriviledged class; Maternal deprivation.

INDEX